manual for

physical agents

fifth edition

manual for physical agents

fifth edition

Karen W. Hayes, PhD, PT

Curriculum Coordinator
Assistant Professor of Physical Therapy
Programs in Physical Therapy
Northwestern University Medical School
Chicago, Illinois

PRENTICE HALL HEALTH
UPPER SADDLE RIVER, NEW JERSEY 07458

Notice: The author and the publisher of this volume have taken care to make certain that the doses of drugs and schedules of treatment are correct and compatible with the standards generally accepted at the time of publication. Nevertheless, as new information becomes available, changes in treatment and in the use of drugs become necessary. The reader is advised to carefully consult the instruction and information material included in the package insert of each drug or therapeutic agent before administration. This advice is especially important when using, administering, or recommending new or infrequently used drugs. The author and publisher disclaim all responsibility for any liability, loss, injury, or damage incurred as a consequence, directly or indirectly, of the use and application of any of the contents of this volume.

www.prenhall.com

05 06 07 08 / 10 9 8 7 6

Prentice Hall International (UK) Limited, *London*
Prentice Hall of Australia Pty. Limited, *Sydney*
Prentice Hall Canada, Inc., *Toronto*
Prentice Hall Hispanoamericana, S.A., *Mexico*
Prentice Hall of India Private Limited, *New Delhi*
Prentice Hall of Japan, Inc., *Tokyo*
Simon & Schuster Asia Pte. Ltd., *Singapore*
Editora Prentice Hall do Brasil Ltda., *Rio de Janeiro*
Prentice Hall, *Upper Saddle River, New Jersey*

Library of Congress Cataloging-in-Publication Data

Hayes, Karen W.
    Manual for physical agents / Karen W. Hayes. — 5th ed.
        p.   cm.
    Includes bibliographical references.
    ISBN 0-8385-6128-4 (pbk. : alk. paper)
        1. Physical therapy Laboratory manuals.   I. Title.
    [RM698.H38   1999]
    615.8'2—dc21   99-22306

Acquisitions Editor: John Butler
Production Editor: Meredith Phillips
Illustrations: ElectraGraphics, Inc.
Designer: Mary Skudlarek

ISBN 0-8385-6128-4
90000

PRINTED IN THE UNITED STATES OF AMERICA

Contributors

Russell A. Foley, MS, PT
Director, Georgia Rehabilitation Center
Newnan, Georgia

Karen W. Hayes, PhD, PT
Curriculum Coordinator
Assistant Professor of Physical Therapy
Programs in Physical Therapy
Northwestern University Medical School
Chicago, Illinois

Wendy Jensen Poe, BS, PT
Senior Clinician of Physical Therapy
Marianjoy/Rehablink
Wheaton, Illinois

Antoinette P. Sander, MS, PT
Instructor in Physical Therapy
Programs in Physical Therapy
Northwestern University Medical School
Chicago, Illinois

Jane Wilding, MS, PT, OCS
Former Assistant Professor of Physical Therapy
Physical Therapy Program
Midwestern University
Downers Grove, Illinois
Currently a graduate student and research assistant in the Doctoral Program in
Kinesiology with specialization in Motor Control at the University of Illinois at Chicago

Contents

Preface

My original motivation for this book was to provide a concise guide to the application of the physical agents for students of physical therapy. Most textbooks at the time did not include instructions about application, and faculty members spent an inordinate amount of time creating written instructions or performing demonstrations. I felt that if students could have instructions complete enough to perform the techniques without prior demonstration, I could spend more time discussing clinical decision making with them.

After students at Northwestern University first used the book, they began to share it with students from other schools, and we began to receive requests for the book. As a result, I worked with a committee of students to obtain specific feedback and make revisions for clarity, and we prepared the book for limited distribution. Since 1975, when the first edition of *Manual for Physical Agents* was published locally by Northwestern University, the book has been adopted by many educational programs for physical therapists, physical therapist assistants, and athletic trainers as a means of helping students apply the many physical agents used in practice.

The manual has been popular for its concise summaries of the theoretical background, step-by-step instructions, generic nature of the instructions, and inclusion of the majority of currently used techniques. Although originally designed as a tool for students, the manual has also enjoyed success among practitioners, serving as a departmental procedural manual and a reminder of how to perform treatments once learned but infrequently practiced. The publication of the fourth edition of this manual marked a new era for the book. With its publication by Appleton & Lange, readers benefited from a more professional presentation and wider availability.

The fifth edition of the book has been thoroughly updated and more heavily referenced. Some chapters on little-used techniques have been eliminated. The chapters on electrical stimulation, traction, and ultrasound have been completely revised. Clinical Tips and additional illustrations have been included throughout the text. As in the past, extensive reading lists have been included to assist the reader in pursuing more information about the agents.

Keeping the manual current through its five editions has been challenging but gratifying. Throughout the years, people too numerous to mention have encouraged me, provided honest criticism, and facilitated the availability of the book. I am especially grateful for the support of Sally C. Edelsberg, Director of Programs in Physical Therapy at Northwestern University; the contributors; the illustrators; and the editors at Appleton & Lange. With this edition, special thanks go to Nicole Hajer, MPT, for her very able assistance and her persistent efforts to keep me on track throughout the revision process.

chapter 1

Guidelines for the Use of Electromedical Equipment

STORAGE

1. Store equipment in a designated area and return it to that area following each use.
2. Coil and store line cords in a safe location.

TREATMENT AREA

1. Obtain wooden plinths that measure 30 × 72 × 30 in. (76.2 × 182.9 × 76.2 cm). Mattresses should *not* contain metal. Supply plenty of pillows that *do not* have zippered covers.
2. Keep an adequate supply of clean linen available.
3. Keep the area clean at all times to reduce the danger of infection. Clean up spilled liquids or paraffin immediately to prevent slipping.
4. Guarantee privacy by using curtains or partitions around each treatment table.
5. Keep electrical cords out of the traffic pattern.
6. Have a fire extinguisher and first aid kit available. Keep them maintained, and know where they are.
7. Set up equipment so that the patient cannot touch it while it is in operation.

ELECTRICAL SAFETY

1. Use only electrical equipment approved by a nationally recognized testing laboratory (e.g., Underwriters' Laboratories).

2. Because of the relatively large amount of electricity drawn by much of the equipment, the area must be equipped with adequate wiring. Each outlet should have a separate 15- to 20-ampere line. To minimize the danger of circuit overloading, check the amount of current drawn by each piece of equipment used. If the amperes are not indicated on the equipment, the watts usually are. Use the formula:

$$\text{amperes} = \text{watts/volts}$$

3. Install ground fault circuit interrupters (GFCIs) in the power receptacles that are within 5 feet (1.5 meters) of a water supply.
4. Check electrical equipment before each use to ensure safe working conditions. Look for frayed wires, breaks in insulation, open switches and connections, and so on. If equipment is not functioning according to expectations, do not use it. Have it repaired immediately.
5. Have all equipment and GFCIs professionally inspected and maintained at least once, preferably twice, a year.
6. Keep water away from electrical equipment.
7. Do not block ventilation of equipment.
8. Avoid using extension cords.
9. Keep patients with cardiac pacemakers isolated from shortwave and microwave diathermies while they are in operation.
10. Use battery-operated devices whenever possible, especially in the home.
11. Always turn all dials to "0" or "OFF" at the end of the treatment.
12. Pull electrical cords from wall receptacles by grasping the plug, not the cord.

READINGS

Berger WH. Electrical shock hazards in the physical therapy department. *Clin Manage Phys Ther.* 1985;5(4):26–31.

Chen D, Mersamma P, Puliyodil PA, Monga TN. Cardiac pacemaker inhibition by transcutaneous electrical nerve stimulation. *Arch Phys Med Rehabil.* 1990;71:27–30.

Ching M, Aston E. Safe use of electromedical equipment. Part I: Mechanisms of electric shock. *Physiother Can.* 1976;28:24–28.

Ching M, Aston E. Safe use of electromedical equipment. Part II: Minimizing electric shock hazards. *Physiother Can.* 1976;28:89–93.

Heath J. The effects of shortwave diathermy, microwave and ultrasonics on demand pacemakers and ventrical inhibited pacemakers. *Aust J Physiother.* 1974;20:144–145.

Jones SL. Electromagnetic field interference and cardiac pacemakers. *Phys Ther.* 1976; 56:1013–1018.

LaBan MM, Petty D, Hauser AM, Taylor RS. Peripheral nerve conduction stimulation: its effect on cardiac pacemakers. *Arch Phys Med Rehabil.* 1988;69:358–362.

Nave CR, Nave BC. *Physics for the Health Sciences.* 2nd ed. Philadelphia: W.B. Saunders; 1980.

Ritter HTM. Instrumentation considerations: operating principles, purchase, management, and safety. In: Michlovitz SL, ed. *Thermal Agents in Rehabilitation.* 3rd ed. Philadelphia: F.A. Davis; 1996:61–77.

Robinson AJ. Instrumentation for electrotherapy. In: Robinson AJ, Snyder-Mackler L, eds. *Clinical Electrophysiology: Electrotherapy and Electrophysiologic Testing.* 2nd ed. Baltimore: Williams & Wilkins; 1995:31–80.

Webber BA. Interference to cardiac pacemakers. *Physiotherapy.* 1975;61:276.

Superficial Heat

Superficial heat may be delivered by a variety of sources, all of which produce electromagnetic waves within the infrared spectrum. Any heated object emits infrared waves, and the wavelength and characteristics of these waves are determined by the temperature of the object. Regardless of how superficial heat is delivered, it penetrates tissues to a depth of only a few millimeters and is absorbed only in the epidermis and dermis. The method of delivery may allow tissues deep to the dermis to be heated through tissue compression and conduction. Superficial heat applications are even capable of increasing intra-articular temperature in joints over which the soft tissue covering is thin; for example, the interphalangeal or knee joints.[1–4]

In this chapter, a general discussion of superficial heat is followed by discussion of the different methods of delivery.

PURPOSE AND EFFECTS

The effects of heat application, including superficial heat application, depend on increasing the temperature of the target tissue to a therapeutic level of 105.8°F to 113°F (41°C to 45°C).[5] This temperature is reached in about 8 to 10 minutes.[6] In response to the heat stimulus, the body produces physiologic responses that may be therapeutic. Within 30 minutes, the body reaches thermal equilibrium, and further heating is not beneficial. The therapeutic effects of superficial heat include:

1. Increased metabolism in the tissues in which heat is absorbed.
2. Increased perspiration in the area of absorption.
3. Linear increase in oxygen tension with increased tissue temperature.[7]
4. Local vasodilatation with hyperemia[6,8] in response to increased demands for nutrients or from stimulation of cells that release a histamine-like substance.

5. Muscle relaxation via effects on the muscle spindles and Golgi tendon organs.[9]
6. Sedation of sensory nerve endings if the heat is mild. At high temperatures, patients do not tolerate moist heat as well as dry heat.[10]
7. Increased capillary pressure and cell permeability, which can promote local swelling.
8. In conjunction with stretching exercises, increased extensibility of connective tissue.[11–14]
9. Increased body temperature and respiratory and pulse rates, as well as decreased blood pressure if applied long enough or systemically. These responses dissipate the excess heat and maintain a thermal equilibrium.

INDICATIONS

1. Subacute and chronic conditions such as osteoarthritis, muscle injury, and muscle tension or guarding.
2. Clean wounds.
3. Stimulation of perspiration to improve electrical conductivity of the skin prior to electrical stimulation.

CONTRAINDICATIONS

1. Acute inflammatory conditions such as sprains and strains may be aggravated by heating.
2. Previously existing fever may be further elevated by systemic heating of the patient.
3. Malignancies may metastasize as a result of the increased blood flow produced by heating.[15]
4. Active bleeding such as that which occurs with acute trauma may be prolonged.
5. Patients with cardiac insufficiency may not be able to tolerate the additional stress on the heart produced by generalized heating.
6. Older adults and children less than 4 years old have unreliable thermoregulatory systems and may develop fever quite easily as a result of generalized heat treatments.
7. Patients with peripheral vascular disease have diminished capacity to meet the increased metabolic demands if tissues in the affected extremities are heated directly. Heating a remote area with the intent of producing a reflex vasodilatation in the skin of the affected extremities is an alternative treatment.[16,17]
8. Tissues that are devitalized by x-ray therapy should not be heated.

PRECAUTIONS

1. With repeated strong doses, undesirable mottled pigmentation may be apparent. This discoloration may result from destruction of red blood cells or paralysis of the arterioles in a dilated state.[18]

2. Previously existing edema may be aggravated by heating. Elevated positions, mild heat intensities, careful observation of skin and tissues, and sequential girth measurements are recommended.
3. Patients with sensory loss may be unreliable judges of heat levels and may also have diminished vascular supplies. If treatment with heat is justifiable, the patient's skin should be carefully observed for excessive redness that may indicate a burn.
4. Patients who are confused are often unreliable judges of heat levels and may not be able to follow safety instructions. These patients should be treated with extreme caution if treated with heat at all.

Radiant Heat

DESCRIPTION

Radiant heat increases the temperature of objects that absorb the infrared waves but does not affect the intervening medium. Two different types of generators, nonluminous and luminous lamps, produce radiant heat. In nonluminous infrared lamps, radiant heat is usually produced by a highly resistant metal (carborundum), much like the element in a toaster. This metal core is housed within a metal reflector. When an electrical current is introduced through the carborundum, its high electrical resistance causes heating and emission of infrared waves. The largest proportion of the emitted waves are long, or far, infrared waves in the range of 3000 to 4000 nm.[19] Short, or near, infrared waves and red visible waves are emitted to a lesser degree (see Appendix A). Consequently, nonluminous lamps are not without the production of light, as the name suggests; rather, they produce a red glow. The power of these nonluminous units may vary from 50 to 1000 watts. The reflector focuses waves to the part being treated and should be covered at its opening with a mesh screen, which protects the patient from injury in the unlikely event that pieces of the carborundum might split off during use. Because of the time necessary to heat the core and generate the maximal output of waves, a warm-up period of 5 to 10 minutes is required.

As an object is heated to higher temperatures, an increasing percentage of the wavelengths emitted are in the short, or near, infrared band. The largest proportion of the waves emitted from luminous generators is in the short infrared range, around 1000 nm.[19] The remainder of the emissions are visible, long infrared, and a small percentage of ultraviolet waves (see Appendix A). Luminous generators are usually tungsten filament light bulbs mounted in metal reflectors. Therefore, luminous lamps, in contrast to nonluminous lamps, produce a bright, white light. The reflector focuses the waves to the part being treated. Power ranges from 60 to 1500 watts. Heat is produced instantly, so no warm-up time is required. Larger bulbs should be separated from the patient by a mesh screen to protect the patient should the bulbs shatter during use.

Long infrared waves are absorbed in the stratum corneum of the epidermis, so they penetrate only 1 to 2 mm. Short infrared and the longer visible waves (>500 nm), which can penetrate up to 10 mm through the epidermis to the dermal layers, are absorbed in all layers of the epidermis and dermis.[6] Because heat is produced where the waves are absorbed, infrared radiation from either source is produced superficially in the skin. Because short infrared waves are absorbed by different layers of the skin, the heat from a luminous generator feels less intense at the same distance than the heat produced by a nonluminous generator whose waves are all absorbed in the same layer of the skin. In addition, because short infrared and visible light waves penetrate slightly more deeply, the short waves can affect nerve endings and vascular beds in the dermis and stimulate more perspiration than the longer wavelengths. The characteristics of long and short infrared waves are summarized in Table 2–1.

ADVANTAGES

1. Radiant heat is useful for seeping wounds that should be dried.
2. Clean wounds are less likely to become infected than they would be if a heat source that contacts the patient were used.
3. The practitioner may visually observe the reactions of the part being treated with infrared radiation.
4. The infrared lamp does not contact the patient, so tenderness is not aggravated.

DISADVANTAGES

1. Because waves spread on leaving the source, treatment of a small, local area with an infrared lamp is difficult.
2. Radiant heat cannot be used if positioning requirements preclude exposure of the body part to be treated. For example, if the posterior aspect is to be heated, and the patient cannot lie in the prone or sidelying position, exposure is impossible.
3. Glare from a luminous lamp can be irritating to the patient's eyes.

TABLE 2–1. Comparison of Long and Short Infrared Waves

INFRARED BAND	WAVELENGTHS	DEPTH OF PENETRATION	TYPE OF LAMP	SKIN–SOURCE DISTANCE	WARM-UP TIME
Long, or far, Infrared	1,500–15,000 nm, especially 3,000–4,000 nm	1–2 mm	Nonluminous	36 in. (91 cm) for 750–1,000 W lamps; 30 in. (76 cm) for 50–600 W lamps	5–10 min
Short, or near, Infrared	800–1,500 nm especially 1,000 nm	Up to 10 mm	Luminous	30 in. (76 cm) for 750–1,000 W lamps; 24 in. (61 cm) for 50–600 W lamps	None

INSTRUCTIONS

1. Check the lamp to see if it is operating, the screen is secure, and the plug is electrically safe. Turn on a nonluminous lamp for 5 to 10 minutes to bring it to operating temperature.
2. Instruct the patient regarding what you are planning to do, what he may expect from treatment, and what you expect of him.
3. Have the patient remove all clothing and jewelry from the area to be treated.
4. Position the patient comfortably so that the area to be treated is accessible.
5. Drape the patient for modesty, leaving the area to be treated uncovered.
6. Check the patient's temperature sensation and the integrity of the skin in the area to be treated.
7. Position the lamp so that the majority of the waves will be perpendicular to the part to be irradiated (see Appendix B, Cosine Law).
8. Remind the patient that he should feel just a comfortable warmth, not as much heat as he can tolerate. Explain that he should not move closer to the lamp or touch the generator, because both acts could cause burns (see Appendix B, Inverse Square Law). Provide a call system, and tell the patient to call if the heat becomes too intense.
9. Adjust the height of the lamp for the appropriate skin source distance, and set a timer for the appropriate amount of treatment time (see below). For safety, when adjusting the height of the lamp, be sure to adjust it away from the patient.
10. If the treatment is given to an area that causes the patient to look at a luminous lamp, protect the patient's eyes from glare and the small amount of ultraviolet radiation, and to prevent overdrying the cornea.
11. Turn on a luminous lamp after the patient is positioned and draped and the distance is measured.
12. Remain nearby to observe the patient's response to treatment.
13. Throughout the treatment, dry any perspiration that forms. Perspiration increases evaporative heat loss and allows the body to reach thermal equilibrium more readily.
14. At the conclusion of the treatment, turn off and remove the lamp. Dry and cover the patient and allow him to rest a few minutes before rising. Return the lamp to its proper location.
15. Perform all appropriate posttreatment evaluations, including checking the skin condition and general physiologic status.
16. Document patient position, area treated, lamp used, distance, duration of treatment, and patient response.

RESPONSES TO TREATMENT AND TREATMENT MODIFICATION

A normal response includes pink skin and perhaps some perspiration. If the patient has very dark skin, changes in skin color may not be observed. If the skin is red or the patient reports excessive heat, move the lamp farther away. If the lamp cannot be moved farther away, a white towel may be placed over the area to reflect some of the incident radiation. Some time after the initiation of treatment, the patient may become accustomed to the heat and request an increase in intensity. Because of this sensory adaptation, however, the patient may not be able to judge a new heat level accurately. Do not lower the lamp to increase the heat; doing so could put the patient at risk for a burn.

If the patient develops very red skin or blisters, turn off the lamp immediately and place a cold or ice pack on the area. File an incident report.

A patient with a strong systemic response to heat may feel dizzy or faint from falling blood pressure. Take the patient's blood pressure and elevate the legs. Monitor blood pressure until it rises to normal levels. Plan milder or more localized treatment in the future.

DOSAGE

Intensity

The skin–source distance determines the intensity of the heat. If using a nonluminous lamp, measure the distance from the highest point on the irradiated surface to the actual heat source (the carborundum core). A large, 750- to 1000-watt, nonluminous generator should be placed 36 in. (91 cm) from the surface to start, and lowered or raised to achieve more or less heat (see Table 2–1). A smaller, 50- to 500-watt lamp may be placed 30 in. (76 cm) away initially. The skin–source distance for a 1000-watt luminous lamp should start at 30 in. (76 cm). For smaller (500- to 600-watt) lamps, start at 24 in. (61 cm) and raise or lower the lamp according to the patient's tolerance. Because shorter infrared waves are absorbed at different depths, distances for luminous lamps may be closer than for nonluminous infrared lamps without danger of producing tissue damage.[5] Generally, mild heating is used with subacute conditions and strong heating with chronic conditions. No treatment should exceed the patient's heat tolerance.

Time

For an initial treatment, subacute conditions, or for preheating prior to electrical stimulation, 15 to 20 minutes is adequate. For chronic conditions, 20 to 30 minutes is recommended.

Frequency

Infrared radiation may be given once or twice daily for subacute conditions and less often for more chronic conditions.

HOME USE

The guidelines in this chapter can be used to instruct patients who are planning to use radiant heat at home. Both heat lamps and sun lamps are available at local pharmacies. Assist patients in choosing a lamp to purchase. Heat lamps are luminous generators and should be used with the same guidelines and precautions that are indicated in this chapter. In the interest of safety, these lamps are usually limited to 250 watts. Some heat lamps contain red bulbs that are less annoying to the eyes and diminish the output of most visible and ultraviolet waves. On the other hand, sun lamps generally have a high proportion of ultraviolet waves. They are not appropriate for use as heat treatments because the time needed to produce the physiologic effects of heat is long enough to cause ultraviolet burns.

Conductive Heat: Hot Packs

DESCRIPTION

Commercial hot packs are a conductive means of delivering moist heat. Some packs are made of canvas and filled with silica gel. They are available in a variety of shapes and sizes and are kept immersed in water of about 170°F (77°C) in a thermostatically controlled heater. These packs are capable of retaining heat for about 10 to 20 minutes.

ADVANTAGES

1. Hot packs are safe in that they become cooler during treatment. Thus, the risk of burning is minimized if enough padding is provided initially.
2. Local areas can be treated effectively with hot packs.

DISADVANTAGES

1. Larger packs can be heavy, and the weight of the pack may aggravate conditions in which tenderness is a problem.
2. Contact with the packs is a potential avenue for infection if an open wound is present.
3. The area treated is not visible, making skin response difficult to monitor.

INSTRUCTIONS

1. Instruct the patient regarding what you are planning to do, what she may expect from treatment, and what you expect of her.
2. Have the patient remove all clothing and jewelry from the area to be treated.
3. Inspect the patient's skin and check temperature sensation in the area to be treated.
4. Position and drape the patient appropriately, comfortably, and modestly. Cover the area to be treated with a clean terry cloth towel. Patients may be positioned to lie on the packs. If so, the practitioner should place the pack before positioning the patient. However, this position compresses the skin and diminishes local circulation. In addition, lying on the bulky pack and padding may be uncomfortable. For patients who cannot lie prone, other positions such as sidelying are preferable.
5. Using the tabs, remove a pack of an appropriate size from the heating unit and place it on a commercial terry cloth cover (Figure 2–1) or on two terry cloth towels folded lengthwise and arranged as illustrated in Figure 2–2.
6. Cover the commercial covers with a moisture-proof, thermal insulating cover. Make sure the tabs are enclosed in the cover. The commercial covers are equivalent to about four to six layers of terry cloth toweling. Add additional layers of toweling so there is the equivalent of six to

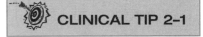

CLINICAL TIP 2–1

Positioning for Hot Packs

When patients are being treated for back problems and cannot lie prone, it is best not to have patients lie on hot packs or heating pads. The patient's weight compresses the skin, diminishing local circulation, and the bulk of the pack and padding may be uncomfortable. Try a sidelying position, and lean the pack against the patient. Use pillows to hold the pack in place or tie the pack on with a strap or sheet.

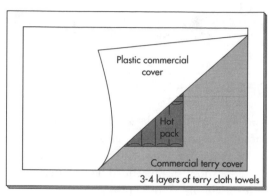

Figure 2-1. Covering the hot pack with the commercial cover.

eight layers of toweling between the pack and the patient. The commercial covers become thin with use, so add additional layers of toweling to compensate as needed. If using towels only to wrap the pack, fold the towels so that six to eight layers of toweling cover the pack (Figure 2–3). If the patient is to lie on the packs, provide more padding to compensate for the diminished local circulation and the compression of the padding from the weight of the patient.

7. Take the pack to the patient and securely place it on the area to be treated. Explain to the patient that the heat should be comfortably warm but not as hot as can be tolerated. Cover the entire area with the sheet or additional dry toweling.

8. Check the patient's reported sensations and skin frequently during the first 5 minutes of treatment. During this time the heat is developing, the pack is hottest, and the patient is at highest risk for a thermal burn. Frequent checks are especially important if the patient is lying on the pack. Make necessary adjustments in padding if the patient is too warm. Provide a call system, and set a timer.

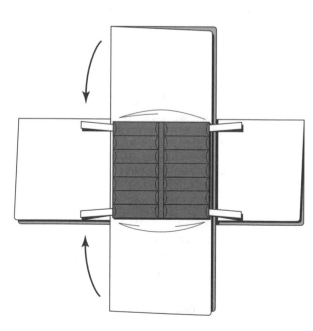

Figure 2-2. Position of towels for wrapping a hot pack.

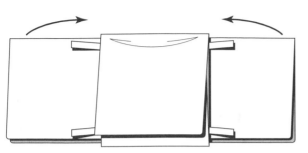

Figure 2-3. Wrapping the hot pack.

9. At the conclusion of the treatment, remove the pack and dry the patient. Check the skin condition and general physiologic response to treatment, and allow her to rest for a few minutes.
10. Return the pack to the heating unit and allow at least one-half hour of reheating before using the pack again.
11. Perform any other appropriate posttreatment evaluation procedures.
12. Document patient position, area treated, size and number of packs, amount of padding, duration of treatment, and patient response.

RESPONSES TO TREATMENT AND TREATMENT MODIFICATION

A normal response includes pink skin and perspiration. If the patient has dark skin, changes in skin color may not be observed. If the skin is red or the patient reports excessive heat, add more towels. If the patient develops very red skin or blisters, remove the pack immediately, and place a cold or ice pack on the area. File an incident report.

DOSAGE

Intensity
The strength of heating is governed by patient tolerance and is accomplished by adding or removing toweling as needed. Hot packs begin to cool after about 10 minutes; if vigorous heating is desired, change the pack and use a fresh one to maintain the thermal gradient.

Time
Duration of treatment is 15 to 30 minutes. If the packs are used for preheating prior to electrical stimulation, a 10- to 15-minute treatment is adequate.

Frequency
Hot packs may be used daily or more often for subacute problems. Frequency may be decreased as the patient improves.

HOME USE

Hot packs are easy to use at home, and there are many ways to make them. The easiest method is purchase of a commercial pack, although these packs involve some expense. These packs can be heated in hot water in a saucepan on the stovetop and wrapped in towels as indicated above. Make sure the patient obtains a thermometer to test the temperature of the water while heating the pack. It should be about 170°F (77°C); the packs should not be boiled. Explain that the method of controlling the heat is to add or remove towels. When commercial packs are not in use, they may be frozen; they should not be allowed to dry.

Some people may have a heating pad at home. Heating pads provide a drier heat than hot packs. Some commercially available heating pads have covers that attract and retain moisture. Because these pads must be hot to be effective, they are not appropriate for patients who require mild-to-moderate heating. Caution patients not to lie on any type of heating pad or to fall asleep using a heating pad. Some heating pads have spring-loaded switches that must be actively held during heating. Releasing the switch, as might occur if a patient fell asleep, causes the pad to cool. Still, it is safest not to fall asleep while using a heating pad.

Microwavable hot packs, which can be heated in a microwave oven, are composed of a material that absorbs heat and moisture. Heating times vary with the power of the oven. Like other hot packs, they stay warm for about 20 minutes. Tell patients to cover these packs with clean toweling before placing them on the skin. These packs mold easily to the contour of the body part.

In all cases, be sure that the patient understands the dosage of superficial heat. Patients may use a hot pack several times a day if they wish, but the heat should not be extremely intense or used for over 30 minutes at a time.

Conductive Heat: Paraffin Bath

DESCRIPTION

A paraffin bath is a tank containing a mixture of medical paraffin and mineral oil (the latter helps lower the melting point). The two ingredients are mixed in a ratio of about 5 lb (2.25 kg) of wax to 1 pt (0.47 L) of oil. The tank may or may not have a built-in heating unit, thermostat, and drain. The paraffin is melted, and the temperature is maintained at 125°F to 127°F (52°C to 53°C). Because of its low specific heat, paraffin is unable to deliver as much heat per gram as water, so the paraffin feels cooler at the same temperature as water. Thus, higher temperatures are necessary to deliver an adequate amount of heat.

ADVANTAGES

1. Paraffin baths are especially useful for the distal extremities.
2. The paraffin-and-oil mixture and the retention of perspiration help soften the skin.

DISADVANTAGES

1. Some patients find the heat level of a paraffin bath excessive. Because the temperature of the bath cannot be lowered without solidifying the wax, mild heat treatments are difficult to deliver.

2. Treatments with liquid paraffin may be messy.
3. Movement must be minimized in a paraffin bath.
4. The tank and paraffin are cumbersome to clean. Refer to the manufacturer's manual for directions.
5. Open wounds in the area requiring treatment should not be immersed in paraffin.
6. Intracapsular heating may promote accelerated destruction of articular cartilage in acute inflammatory joint pathologies.[20]

INSTRUCTIONS

There are several methods of delivering a paraffin bath. The three most useful are discussed below. The immersion bath produces the greatest increase in skin temperature.[21] The dip-immersion method is not as effective as the immersion method for raising skin temperature but may be more easily tolerated. Although the glove method is the safest and most commonly used of the three techniques, it is the least effective for raising skin temperature.

1. Instruct the patient regarding what you are planning to do, what he may expect from treatment, and what you expect of him.
2. Check the temperature of the bath to be certain it is 125°F to 127°F (52°C to 53°C).
3. Wash the part to be treated and check it for temperature sensation and skin integrity.
4. Position the patient comfortably, and drape the patient carefully to keep paraffin from soiling clothes.
5. Immerse the part to be treated in the bath, and instruct the patient to avoid movement that would crack the solid layer of paraffin that builds up because the skin temperature is lower than that of the paraffin. Warn him not to touch the bottom of the tank.

Immersion Bath

In an immersion bath, the patient holds the part in the bath for the duration of the treatment.

Dip Immersion

Instruct the patient to dip and remove the part once or twice and allow the paraffin on the part to harden. Then immerse the part as for an immersion bath. This hardened layer partially insulates the skin, so the temperature is more comfortable.

Glove

Before immersing the part, obtain waxed paper, plastic wrap or a plastic bag, and rubber bands or tape. Set aside two terry cloth towels that have been folded lengthwise. Instruct the patient to dip the part, remove it, and allow the paraffin on the part to harden until it looks dull. Repeat this process 6 to 12 times so that a glove of solid paraffin is formed. After the last dip has hardened, quickly wrap the part with the paraffin glove in the paper, plastic, or bag, and then in several layers of the terry cloth toweling. Secure with the rubber bands or tape. Thick insulation on all surfaces optimizes heat retention. Be sure to close off all avenues of heat escape.

6. At the conclusion of the treatment, remove the part and let the liquid paraffin harden. Remove the paraffin from the part by peeling it off or by having the patient perform active exercises to cause it to crack.

7. If the patient is to receive a massage, do it at this time. If not, clean and dry the part.

8. Perform all appropriate posttreatment evaluation procedures, including checking skin condition and general physiologic response.

9. Dry the perspiration from the solid paraffin with clean paper towels. Some clinics return the paraffin to the tank. At the end of the day, a heating circuit can be activated to raise the temperature of the tank sufficiently to kill any bacteria. The temperature stabilizes at the proper level by the next morning. Other clinics dispose of used paraffin and periodically add fresh paraffin and oil to the tank. Dispose of paraffin carefully because it is highly flammable.

10. Document patient position; area treated; method of treatment, including number of layers if the glove method is used; temperature of the paraffin; duration of treatment; and patient response.

RESPONSES TO TREATMENT AND TREATMENT MODIFICATION

A patient who responds normally has pink, oily skin and perspiration. It is difficult to observe the skin during treatment and color changes may not be noticed with very dark skin, so if the patient reports excessive heat, try adding some insulation by forming separate layers of wax using the dip technique. If the patient is still uncomfortable, terminate the treatment. If the patient has developed very red skin or blisters, place a cold or ice pack on the area. File an incident report.

DOSAGE

Intensity
The amount of heat in a paraffin treatment is determined by the method. The immersion method is most intense, followed by the dip-immersion method. The glove method is least intense and is most appropriate for very mild heating.

Time
Duration of treatment is usually 20 minutes.

Frequency
A paraffin bath is given daily for subacute problems or less often for more chronic conditions.

HOME USE

Small commercial paraffin baths are available. Instruct the patient in their use according to the selected technique and the above instructions. Other methods of

---

CLINICAL TIP 2-2

Cleaning the Paraffin Bath

To keep the paraffin bath clean, be sure to remove any debris before returning used paraffin to the bath. After treatments, use the thermostatic control to increase the bath temperature to over 200°F (93.3°C) and kill any bacteria present. Sediment accumulates over time. After about 6 months of regular use, drain the bath and dispose of the soiled paraffin with other hazardous waste.

home treatment with paraffin have been used such as roasters, crock pots, and sauce pots. Discourage the use of these methods because paraffin is highly flammable. If the treatment is worth using at home, the relatively small investment in a home unit is justified.

Be sure to provide the patient with information about how to obtain medical paraffin and how much oil to add. The patient must understand that the paraffin used for home canning is inappropriate for treatment. It has a higher melting point and would be excessively hot. Because of its flammability, instruct the patient to dispose of used paraffin by taking it to a hazardous waste disposal center.

Conductive Heat: Fluidotherapy

DESCRIPTION

Fluidotherapy is a means of providing dry superficial heat that uses very fine cellulose particles through which heated air is blown. The particles are contained in a tank that has access portals in the top and sides for the extremities (Figure 2–4). The portals are provided with a fine mesh sleeve that closes snugly around the extremity to prevent the particles from being blown into the environment. Three sizes of tanks are available for clinical use; a small one appropriate for single extremity treatment, one that can be used for bilateral upper or lower extremity treatment, and a large unit that can accommodate an entire lower extremity. With Fluidotherapy, the specific heat is lower than that of water, so treatments are delivered at 105°F to 125°F (41°C to 52°C). There are low and high air speeds, and the air may be pulsed through the particles if desired.

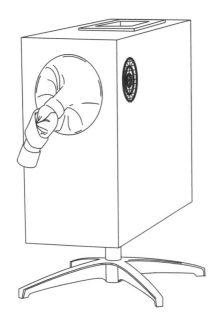

Figure 2-4. Fluidotherapy unit, showing top and side portals.

ADVANTAGES

1. The patient can move during treatment, and practitioners may enter the unit through unused portals to exercise the patient during treatment.
2. The air pressure ostensibly prevents local swelling that occurs when using heat in a dependent position.
3. The particles can be sterilized in the unit and thus do not need replacement.
4. Temperature is maintained at a constant level through a thermostat; the medium does not cool during treatment.
5. Fluidotherapy can be used for wound management if the wound is covered with a dressing or contained in a plastic bag to keep the particles from contacting the wound surface.[22]
6. The moving particles eliminate temperature gradients and serve to re-stimulate the skin receptors so there is less sensory adaptation than with other static heat treatments.

DISADVANTAGES

1. In spite of efforts to contain the particles, some manage to escape and can be very slippery. Be sure to sweep the floor after use.
2. The part to be treated can be lifted from the particles, but it is less visible for observation compared with radiant heat treatments.

INSTRUCTIONS

1. Check the unit to see if it is operating, the sleeves are closed, and the plug is electrically safe. Preheat the unit to the treatment temperature. Preheating usually takes about 45 minutes. For this reason, it is best to preheat the unit in advance of the patient's appointment time.
2. Instruct the patient regarding what you are planning to do, what she may expect from treatment, and what you expect of her.
3. Have the patient remove all clothing and jewelry from the area to be treated.
4. Check the patient's temperature sensation and the integrity of the skin in the area to be treated.
5. Position the patient comfortably so that the area to be treated is accessible, and the patient is able to enter the unit comfortably. If the top openings are to be used for lower extremity treatment, seat the patient above the unit.
6. Drape the patient for modesty and to protect the clothing from the few particles that escape or adhere to the skin, but leave the area to be treated uncovered.
7. Have the patient place her arm(s) or leg(s) in the appropriate opening(s). Either side or top openings are useful for upper extremities. The top openings are more easily used for lower extremities.

8. Secure the straps around the access sleeves to minimize particle escape. Be careful not to strap the patient so tightly that the strap becomes a tourniquet.
9. Check the temperature and if correct, turn on the blower.
10. Remind the patient that she should feel just a comfortable warmth, not as much heat as she can tolerate. Provide a call system, and tell the patient to call if the heat becomes too intense.
11. Remain nearby to observe the patient's response to treatment.
12. At the conclusion of the treatment, turn off the blower. Shake the particles from the sleeves, and then carefully open the sleeves and brush the particles from the patient's skin. Allow the patient to rest a few minutes before moving about. Return the unit to its proper location.
13. Perform all appropriate posttreatment evaluations, including checking the skin condition and general physiologic status.
14. Document patient position, area treated, temperature, duration of treatment, and patient response.

RESPONSES TO TREATMENT AND TREATMENT MODIFICATION

A normal response includes pink skin and perhaps some perspiration. If the patient has very dark skin, changes in skin color may not be observed. If the patient reports excessive heat and the skin is red, terminate the treatment. The unit takes 20 minutes to cool, which is too slow for readjustment of the temperature during treatment. If the patient develops very red skin or blisters, place a cold or ice pack on the area. File an incident report.

DOSAGE

Intensity
Treatments are delivered at 105°F to 125°F (41°C to 52°C).

Time
For an initial treatment or subacute conditions, a 20-minute treatment is adequate. For chronic problems, a 20- to 30-minute treatment is recommended.

Frequency
Treatments may be delivered daily for subacute conditions or less frequently for chronic conditions.

HOME USE

A small Fluidotherapy unit, with one top and one side portal, is available for home use. If deemed appropriate for the patient, instruct the patient in its use according to the directions above.

REFERENCES

1. Hollander JL, Horvath SM. The influence of physical therapy procedures on the intra-articular temperature of normal and arthritic subjects. *Am J Med Sci.* 1949;218:543–548.
2. Oosterveld FGJ, Rasker JJ. Effects of local heat and cold treatment on surface and articular temperature of arthritic knees. *Arthritis Rheum.* 1994;37:1578–1582.
3. Oosterveld FGJ, Rasker JJ, Jacobs JWG, Overmars HJA. The effect of local heat and cold therapy on the intra-articular and skin surface temperature of the knee. *Arthritis Rheum.* 1992;35:146–151.
4. Weinberger A, Fadilah R, Lev A, Pinkhas J. Intra-articular temperature measurements after superficial heating. *Scand J Rehabil Med.* 1989;21:55–57.
5. Lehmann JF, DeLateur BJ. Therapeutic heat. In: Lehmann JF, ed. *Therapeutic Heat and Cold.* 3rd ed. Baltimore: Williams & Wilkins; 1982.
6. Lehmann JF, Silverman DR, Baum BA, et al. Temperature distributions in the human thigh, produced by infared, hot pack and microwave applications. *Arch Phys Med Rehabil.* 1966;47:291–299.
7. Rabkin JM, Hunt TK. Local heat increases blood flow and oxygen tension in wounds. *Arch Surg.* 1987;122:221–225.
8. McMeeken J. Tissue temperature and blood flow: a research based overview of electrophysical modalities. *Aust J Physiother.* 1994;40:49–57.
9. Mense S. Effects of temperature on the discharge of muscle spindles and tendon organs. *Pflügers Arch.* 1978;374:159–166.
10. Abramson DI, Tuck S, Lee SW, et al. Comparison of wet and dry heat in raising temperature of tissues. *Arch Phys Med Rehabil.* 1967;48:654–661.
11. Lehmann JF, Masock AJ, Warren CG, Koblanski JN. Effect of therapeutic temperatures on tendon extensibility. *Arch Phys Med Rehabil.* 1970;51:481–487.
12. Lentell G, Hetherington T, Eagan J, Morgan M. The use of thermal agents to influence the effectiveness of a low-load prolonged stretch. *J Orthop Sports Phys Ther.* 1992;16:200–207.
13. Prentice WE. An electromyographic analysis of the effectiveness of heat or cold and stretching for inducing relaxation in injured muscle. *J Orthop Sports Phys Ther.* 1982;3:133–140.
14. Warren CG, Lehmann JF, Koblanski JN. Heat and stretch procedures: an evaluation using rat tail tendon. *Arch Phys Med Rehabil.* 1976;57:122–126.
15. Sicard-Rosenbaum L, Danoff JV, Guthrie JA, Eckhaus MA. Effects of energy-matched pulsed and continuous ultrasound on tumor growth in mice. *Phys Ther.* 1998;78:271–277.
16. Abramson DI, Tuck S, Chu LSW, et al. Indirect vasodilatation in thermotherapy. *Arch Phys Med Rehabil.* 1965;46:412–420.
17. Wessman HC, Kottke FJ. The effect of indirect heating on peripheral blood flow, pulse rate, blood pressure, and temperature. *Arch Phys Med Rehabil.* 1967;48:567–576.
18. Scott PM. *Clayton's Electrotherapy and Actinotherapy.* 7th ed. Baltimore: Williams & Wilkins; 1975.
19. Low J, Bazin S, Docker M, et al. Guidelines for the safe use of infra-red and radiant heat therapy. *Physiotherapy.* 1992;78:499–500.
20. Harris ED, McCroskery PA. The influence of temperature and fibril stability on degradation of cartilage collagen by rheumatoid synovial collagenase. *N Engl J Med.* 1974;290:1–6.
21. Stimson CW, Rose GB, Nelson PA. Paraffin bath as thermotherapy: an evaluation. *Arch Phys Med Rehabil.* 1958;39:219–227.
22. Valenza J, Rossi C, Parker R, Henley EJ. A clinical study of a new heat modality: fluidotherapy. *J Am Pod Assoc.* 1979;69:440–442.

ADDITIONAL READINGS

Physiology of Superficial Heat

Cornwall MW. Effect of temperature on muscle force and rate of muscle force production in men and women. *J Orthop Sports Phys Ther.* 1994;20:74–80.

Downey JA, Darling RC, Miller JM. The effects of heat, cold, and exercise on the peripheral circulation. *Arch Phys Med Rehabil.* 1968;49:308–314.

Henricson AS, Fredriksson K, Persson I, et al. The effect of heat and stretching on the range of motion of the hip. *J Orthop Sports Phys Ther.* 1984;6:110–115.

Wright V, Johns RJ. Quantitative and qualitative analysis of joint stiffness in normal subjects and in patients with connective tissue diseases. *Ann Rheum Dis.* 1961;20:36–46.

Radiant Heat

Currier DP, Kramer JF. Sensory nerve conduction: heating effects of ultrasound and infrared. *Physiother Can.* 1982;34:241–246.

Hamilton DE, Bywaters EGL, Please NW. A controlled trial of various forms of physiotherapy in arthritis. *Br Med J.* 1959;1:542–544.

Lehmann JF, Brunner GD, Stow RW. Pain threshold measurements after therapeutic application of ultrasound, microwaves and infrared. *Arch Phys Med Rehabil.* 1958;39:560–565.

Montgomery PC. The compounding effects of infrared and ultraviolet irradiation upon normal human skin. *Phys Ther.* 1973;53:489–496.

Sweeney FX, Horvath SM, Mellette HC, Hutt BK. Infrared heating of tissues. *Arch Phys Med Rehabil.* 1950;31:493–501.

Hot Packs

Fyfe M. Skin temperature, color and warmth felt in Hydrocollator pack applications to the lumbar region. *Aust J Physiother.* 1982;28:12–15.

Greenberg R. Effects of hot packs and exercise on local blood flow. *Phys Ther.* 1972;52:273–278.

Hecht PJ, Bachmann S, Booth RE, Rothman RH. Effects of thermal therapy on rehabilitation after total knee arthroplasty. *Clin Orthop.* 1983;178:198–201.

McCay RE, Patton NJ. Pain relief of trigger points: a comparison of moist heat and shortwave diathermy. *J Orthop Sports Phys Ther.* 1984;5:175–178.

Paraffin Bath

Bromley J, Unsworth A, Haslock I. Changes in stiffness following short- and long-term application of standard physiotherapeutic techniques. *Br J Rheumatol.* 1994;33:555–561.

Burns SP, Conin TA. The use of paraffin wax in the treatment of burns. *Physiother Can.* 1987;39:258–260.

Dellhag B, Wollersjö I, Bjelle A. Effect of active hand exercise and wax bath treatment in rheumatoid arthritis patients. *Arthritis Care Res.* 1992;5:87–92.

Hamilton DE, Bywaters EGL, Please NW. A controlled trial of various forms of physiotherapy in arthritis. *Br Med J.* 1959;1:542–544.

Harris R, Millard JB. Paraffin-wax baths in the treatment of rheumatoid arthritis. *Ann Rheum Dis.* 1955;14:278–282.

Hoyrup G, Kjorvel L. Comparison of whirlpool and wax treatments for hand therapy. *Physiother Can.* 1986;38:79–82.

Fluidotherapy

Alcorn R, Bowser B, Henley EJ, Holloway V. Fluidotherapy and exercise in the management of sickle cell anemia: a clinical report. *Phys Ther.* 1984;64:1520–1522.

Borrell RM, Henley EJ, Ho P, Hubbell MK. Fluidotherapy: evaluation of a new heat modality. *Arch Phys Med Rehabil.* 1977;58:69–71.

Borrell RM, Parker R, Henley EJ, et al. Comparison of in vivo temperatures produced by hydrotherapy, paraffin wax treatment, and Fluidotherapy. *Phys Ther.* 1980;60:1273–1276.

Comparisons of Superficial Heat With Other Agents

Halliday Pegg SM, Littler TR, Littler EN. A trial of ice therapy and exercise in chronic arthritis. *Physiotherapy.* 1969;55:51–56.

Hawkes J, Care G, Dixon JS, et al. Comparison of three physiotherapy regimens for hands with rheumatoid arthritis. *Br Med J.* 1985;291:1016.

Kirk JA, Kersley GD. Heat and cold in the physical treatment of rheumatoid arthritis of the knee. *Ann Phys Med.* 1968;9:270–274.

Landen BR. Heat or cold for the relief of low back pain? *Phys Ther.* 1967;47:1126–1128.

Williams J, Harvey J, Tennenbaum H. Use of superficial heat versus ice for the rheumatoid arthritic shoulder: a pilot study. *Physiother Can.* 1986;38:8–13.

3

Hydrotherapy

WATER AS A MEDIUM FOR EXERCISE

Due to certain of its physical properties, water can be used advantageously as a medium for exercise. It is beyond the scope of this book to discuss the exercise management of patients in a therapeutic pool, but an understanding of the principles of underwater exercise may enhance the effectiveness of treatment in a whirlpool or Hubbard tank.

One of the properties of water, buoyancy, contributes to producing a gravity-eliminated environment for the patient. Archimedes' Principle states that an immersed object experiences an upward thrust equal to the weight of the water displaced. Thus, the weight of the patient is supported in water; upward movement is assisted, and downward movement is resisted.

The specific gravity of an object is a measure of its density in grams per cubic centimeter. The specific gravity of water is taken as 1.00 g/cm^3. Due to the buoyancy of the water, any object with a specific gravity of less than 1.00 g/cm^3 floats, whereas objects with specific gravity greater than 1.00 g/cm^3 sink. The specific gravity of the human body with inflated lungs is 0.974 g/cm^3.[1] Therefore, the body floats. The combination of specific gravity and buoyancy renders a patient essentially weightless.

Another property of water that affects movement through it is viscosity. Because of the cohesive forces between molecules, liquids tend to resist flow. This resistance to flow is known as viscosity and varies with different liquids. Viscosity serves to resist movement through the water in all directions, with increasing resistance offered at higher speeds of movement.

To summarize, in a water environment, slow movement in an upward direction is easiest because it is assisted by the buoyancy of the water. Movements parallel to the surface of the water are slightly more difficult, especially if they are performed quickly. The buoyancy supports the weight of the part, and the viscosity resists the movement. The most difficult movement in water is movement in a downward direction. Buoyancy resists downward movement, and, if the movement is fast, viscosity resists it as well.

Whirlpool

DESCRIPTION

A whirlpool is a water bath in which the water is agitated by an electric turbine. Whirlpools, which are made of stainless steel or acrylic material, come in various shapes and sizes, but they all work on the same principles. Although whirlpools can be used for both heating and cooling, their use for heating is discussed here.

PURPOSE AND EFFECTS

A whirlpool is a source of moist heat, delivered by conduction and convection. As with other agents that heat by conduction, subcutaneous tissues may be heated by conduction from adjacent tissue layers. The effects produced by superficial heat are reviewed in Chapter 2. In addition to the heating effects, water produces hydrostatic pressure, an inward pressure exerted against the part being treated. This pressure increases with greater depth and tends to increase the rate of flow in the lymphatic vessels. The hydrostatic pressure may work to minimize any edema that would be produced by heat, although venous congestion and edema continue to occur.[2,3]

The combination of the moist medium and agitation may assist in cleansing stage III and IV wounds and burns and preparing them for débridement. In addition, the combination assists affected patients with mobility activities after hydrotherapy.[4,5] The agitation in a whirlpool can serve several purposes.

1. It provides phasic stimuli to the skin afferents, continuously reactivating them. Thus, the warm water continues to feel warm throughout the treatment.
2. It increases hydrostatic pressure, which may increase lymphatic circulation.
3. It provides a means of grading exercise. The patient can move a limb either with the turbulence to provide assistance for movement or against the adjustable turbulence to increase resistance slightly or greatly.
4. It decreases the thermal gradients within the water, keeping the temperature of the water within the tank consistent throughout.
5. It can remove debris and necrotic tissue from wounds and decrease the bacterial load.[6]

ADVANTAGES

1. The part is visible during treatment.
2. Good dosage control is available.

3. Large tissue temperature increases can be produced, because the part is insulated from evaporative heat loss.
4. Wounds that may be present are not at risk of injury during the transfer of heat and may be cleansed.
5. The patient can move safely during treatment, making the patient more comfortable and allowing the patient to elongate structures while they are heated.

DISADVANTAGES

1. The part to be treated must be in a dependent position.
2. The treatment is costly to install, maintain, operate, and supervise.

INDICATIONS

1. Stage III and IV wounds and burns.[5]
2. Subacute or chronic traumatic or inflammatory conditions. Adjust the water temperature according to the acuity of the condition.
3. Early peripheral vascular disease. Avoid high water temperatures.
4. Peripheral nerve injuries and other conditions that produce muscle weakness.

CONTRAINDICATIONS

All the contraindications listed for superficial heat apply to the use of hydrotherapy as a heating agent. In addition, venous ulcers should not be treated with hydrotherapy because of the risk of venous congestion.[7]

PRECAUTIONS

All the precautions listed for superficial heat apply to the use of hydrotherapy as a heating agent. Other precautions include:

1. When body temperature equals environmental temperature, the only means of heat loss is evaporation. If a large proportion of the patient is immersed in water, the remaining skin surface may not be sufficient for adequate heat loss, and faintness or fever may develop. Keep the room humidity low or provide cold compresses to the head and a cool drink. Treatment should be terminated if necessary.
2. Occasionally, a patient may become "seasick" from watching the water, especially if they are anxious or overly warm. Consider draping the tank.
3. Be certain that the hydrotherapy area is equipped with ground fault circuit interrupters.

INSTRUCTIONS

1. Fill the tank with water of the desired temperature.
2. If open wounds are present, add a disinfectant to the water such as povidone-iodine or sodium hypochlorite.

3. The treatment room should be comfortably warm, well ventilated without being drafty, and with low humidity.

4. Instruct the patient regarding what to expect and what you expect of her.

5. Allow the patient to undress and provide her with suitable garments such as drawstring shorts or a bathing suit.

6. Place a chair by the side of the whirlpool for treatment of the upper extremity, a high seat at the end of the whirlpool for a foot or ankle treatment, or a seat in the whirlpool for more general treatments.

7. Position the patient so that the area to be treated is in the water and the patient is comfortably supported. Use dry padding at the rim of the tank to prevent impairment of circulation and to provide for maximal comfort.

8. If dressings are present, remove them or allow them to soak off before turning on the agitator.

9. The turbine ejector (Figure 3–1) must be kept open at all times. The ejector is cooled by the water in the tank circulating around it at a rate of up to 45 gal/min. To ensure free circulation of the water, check the following:

    a. The small hole at the bottom of the shaft must be at least 2 in. (5 cm) below the surface of the water at all times when the turbine is running.

    b. The patient must not lean against or place fingers and toes against the ejector.

    c. No dressings or hospital gowns should be floating in the water, because they can be sucked into the turbine.

10. The agitation may be adjusted for force, aeration, direction, and depth.

    a. The throttle near the top of the shaft adjusts the force of the agitation.

    b. The butterfly knob near the top of the shaft adjusts the aeration.

    c. The entire unit moves from side to side.

    d. The knob on the suspension bracket at the back of the unit releases the shaft and permits it to be raised and lowered. Make adjustments in height with the agitator turned off.

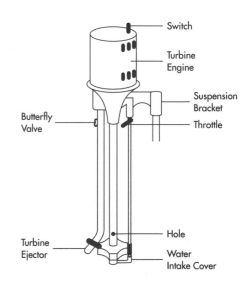

Figure 3–1. Parts of the turbine.

11. Direct the turbulence at the involved area unless it causes additional pain. If so, indirect agitation may be used. Turbulence should be gentle at first and increased according to patient tolerance.
12. An attendant should be present or nearby throughout the treatment.
13. At the conclusion of the treatment, dry the patient and provide dry clothing if necessary. Allow the patient to rest unless she is to receive a massage or local exercise to elongate heated structures. If the position of the patient in the whirlpool requires that the part be in a dependent position, which can encourage edema in the distal segments, have the patient exercise throughout the treatment and elevate the part following treatment.
14. Perform all indicated posttreatment evaluations, including checking skin condition and general physiologic status.
15. Document the temperature and duration of treatment, direction and force of the agitation, and patient response.

DOSAGE

Intensity

Table 3–1 lists the usual temperature ranges.

1. Patients with open wounds, circulatory disorders, and cardiac conditions should receive neutral to warm baths, depending on the extent and severity of the condition.
2. Patients with chronic problems may receive hotter baths than patients with more acute problems.
3. Patients with small local areas to be treated may be treated with warmer temperatures than patients with generalized conditions. Temperatures for full-body immersions should not exceed 102°F (39°C).
4. Patients with painful conditions, if no other contraindicated condition exists, may receive hot to very hot baths.
5. Patients who receive the whirlpool treatment solely as a medium for exercise should receive tepid baths. Temperatures higher than those in the tepid range produce fatigue.[1]

TABLE 3–1. Common Temperature Ranges Used With Hydrotherapy

DESCRIPTOR	°F	°C*
Very hot	104.0–110.0	40.0–43.5
Hot	99.0–104.0	37.0–40.0
Warm	96.0–99.0	35.5–37.0
Neutral	92.0–96.0	33.5–35.5
Tepid	80.0–92.0	27.0–33.5

* Degrees Celcius are rounded to the nearest half degree.

6. Exceeding 110°F (43°C) is not safe or necessary with any whirlpool treatment.

Duration

The duration of the treatment should be about 20 minutes depending on patient tolerance.

Frequency

Whirlpool treatments may be given daily or twice daily for acute problems and less often for more chronic ones.

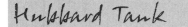

Hubbard Tank

DESCRIPTION

The Hubbard tank is a butterfly-shaped whirlpool in which a patient may be recumbent (Figure 3–2). It is designed so that the patient can move his extremities through abduction movements while the practitioner is able to assist physically from outside the tank. Most Hubbard tanks are equipped with a stretcher that may be fitted into an adjustable support bracket. Two agitators are mounted on a track that allows their position to be modified. To facilitate transfer in and out of the tank, a one-quarter ton electric hoist should be installed on a track over the tank.

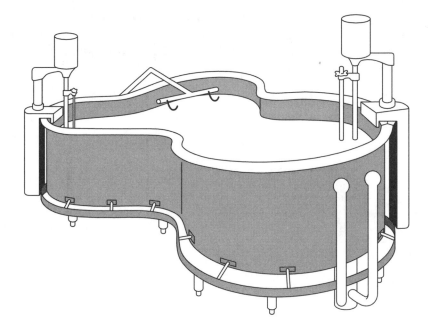

Figure 3–2. The Hubbard tank.

PURPOSE AND EFFECTS

The primary purpose of the Hubbard tank is to deliver heat or cold to a large part of the body. A second purpose is to allow a patient to exercise in an environment that supports the weight of the body or body part.

ADVANTAGES

1. Using a Hubbard tank may prove advantageous for the patient who cannot or should not assume a sitting position or who has difficulty in transferring.
2. Exercises may be performed in the tank.

DISADVANTAGE

Due to installation, maintenance, and operating costs, Hubbartd tank treatments are necessarily expensive and should be used only if a smaller tank will not accomplish the same purpose.

INDICATIONS

1. Generalized wounds such as stage III or IV wounds or burns.
2. Generalized painful conditions.
3. General sedation or relaxation.

CONTRAINDICATIONS

Refer to those listed for whirlpool.

PRECAUTIONS

1. Because so much of a patient's body is immersed in a Hubbard tank, the temperature of the water should not exceed 102°F (39°C), and the patient's vital signs should be observed closely. If the patient becomes flushed or perspires heavily, record the vital signs. If blood pressure falls, body temperature rises, or heart rate increases substantially, terminate treatment.
2. Because warm water is so relaxing, patients who are incontinent may void during treatment.

INSTRUCTIONS

1. The treatment room should be warm with low humidity. Fill the tank with water of an appropriate temperature.

2. Instruct the patient as to what to expect and what you expect of him. The patient should undress and be provided with a bathing suit or similar garment. Hospital gowns are unsatisfactory, because the agitation causes the gown to float, leaving the patient exposed.

3. Check the patient's temperature sensation, skin integrity, and vital signs.

4. Position the stretcher on a plinth next to the tank. Place a strap in a position to go around the stretcher and the patient. Provide a waterproof pillow.

5. Have the patient lie on the plinth with his weight evenly distributed, and secure the strap.

6. Attach the hoist to the rings on the four corners of the stretcher.

7. Raise the hoist, thus lifting the patient, swing him over the tank, and lower him to just above the water level. DO NOT ALLOW THE PATIENT TO OPERATE THE HOIST.

8. Attach the head end of the stretcher to the support bracket.

9. Allow the patient to test the water with his hand, if desired, before lowering the patient into the water until the stretcher rests on the bottom of the tank. Remove the hoist.

10. Adjust the agitators to direct the agitation toward the site of involvement.

11. Monitor the patient's physiologic responses throughout treatment.

12. To remove the patient, reattach the hoist, raise the stretcher to above the water line, and tipping the stretcher slightly, allow its hollow tubing to drain.

13. Cover the patient with dry bath blanketing, and remove wet garments, if possible.

14. Raise the hoist high enough to clear the side of the tank, and swing the patient on the stretcher over to the plinth. Lower the patient to the plinth and remove the hoist.

15. Dry the patient quickly and thoroughly.

16. Perform all indicated posttreatment evaluations, including measurement of vital signs.

17. Document the temperature and duration of treatment, direction and amount of agitation, and patient response.

DOSAGE

Intensity

Hubbard tank treatments should not exceed 102°F (39°C).

Duration

Hubbard tank treatments should be limited to about 20 minutes. Treatments for burns may be longer, but if no electrolytes have been added to the water, 30 minutes is the maximum to avoid leaching of the patient's electrolytes.

Frequency

The Hubbard tank can be used for acute or subacute problems as often as twice a day and less often for more chronic conditions.

CLINICAL TIP 3–1

Cleaning and Disinfecting Hydrotherapy Equipment

Clean the whirlpool or Hubbard tank with a phenolic germicidal detergent,[8] paying special attention to the ejector, thermometer shaft, seams, and drain, and then rinse thoroughly. Cleaning solutions should be obtained after discussion with the housekeeping and microbiology departments. Have bacterial colony counts run on the equipment on a random basis at least once per month.

REFERENCES

1. Scott PM. *Clayton's Electrotherapy and Actinotherapy.* 7th ed. Baltimore: Williams & Wilkins; 1975.
2. Magness JL, Garrett TR, Erickson DJ. Swelling of the upper extremity during whirlpool baths. *Arch Phys Med Rehabil.* 1970;51:297–299.
3. McCulloch JM, Boyd VB. The effects of whirlpool and the dependent position on lower extremity volume. *J Orthop Sports Phys Ther.* 1992;16:169–173.
4. Mulder GD, Brazinsky BA, Seeley JE. Factors complicating wound repair. In: McCulloch JM, Kloth LC, Feedar JA, eds. *Wound Healing: Alternatives in Management.* 2nd ed. Philadelphia: F. A. Davis; 1995.
5. Feedar JA. Clinical management of chronic wounds. In: McCulloch JM, Kloth LC, Feedar JA, eds. *Wound Healing: Alternatives in Management.* 2nd ed. Philadelphia: F. A. Davis; 1995.
6. Bohannon RW. Whirlpool versus whirlpool and rinse for removal of bacteria from a venous stasis ulcer. *Phys Ther.* 1982;62:304–308.
7. McCulloch JM. Treatment of wounds caused by vascular insufficiency. In: McCulloch JM, Kloth LC, Feedar JA, eds. *Wound Healing: Alternatives in Management.* 2nd ed. Philadelphia: F. A. Davis; 1995.
8. Harkess N. Bacteriology. In: McCulloch JM, Kloth LC, Feedar JA, eds. *Wound Healing: Alternatives in Management.* 2nd ed. Philadelphia: F. A. Davis; 1995.

ADDITIONAL READINGS

General

Borrell RM, Parker R, Henley EJ, et al. Comparison of in vivo temperatures produced by hydrotherapy, paraffin wax treatment, and Fluidotherapy. *Phys Ther.* 1980;60:1273–1276.

Coté DJ, Prentice WE, Hooker DN, Shields EW. Comparison of three treatment procedures for minimizing ankle sprain swelling. *Phys Ther.* 1988;68:1072–1076.

Hoyrup G, Kjorvel L. Comparison of whirlpool and wax treatments for hand therapy. *Physiother Can.* 1986;38:79–82.

Toomey R, Grief-Schwartz R. Extent of whirlpool use in Canadian physiotherapy departments: a survey. *Physiother Can.* 1986;38:277–278.

Toomey R, Grief-Schwartz R, Piper MC. Clinical evaluation of the effects of whirlpool on patients with Colles' fractures. *Physiother Can.* 1986;38:280–284.

Water as a Medium for Exercise

Goldby LJ, Scott DL. The way forward for hydrotherapy. *Br J Rheumatol.* 1993;32:771–773.

Hall J, Skevington SM, Maddison PJ, Chapman K. A randomized and controlled trial of hydrotherapy in rheumatoid arthritis. *Arthritis Care Res.* 1996;9:206–215.

Roberts J, Freeman J. Hydrotherapy management of low back pain: a quality improvement project. *Aust J Physiol.* 1995;41:205–208.

Wound Care

Gogia PP, Hirt BS, Zirn TT. Wound management with whirlpool and infrared cold laser treatment: a clinical report. *Phys Ther.* 1988;68:1239–1242.

Headley B, Robson MC, Krizek TJ. Methods of reducing environmental stress for the acute burn patient. *Phys Ther.* 1975;55:5–9.

Niederhuber SS, Stribley RF, Koepke GH. Reduction of skin bacterial load with use of the therapeutic whirlpool. *Phys Ther.* 1975;55:482–486.

Richard RL, Finley RK, Miller SF. Effect of hydrotherapy on burn wound bacteria [abstract R-182]. *Phys Ther.* 1984;64:46.

Cleaning

Grabois M, Wiechec F, Zislis J. Sterilization of Hubbard tank units with povidone-iodine and Ampro pool filter. *Arch Phys Med Rehabil.* 1973;54:441–443.

Highsmith AK, Kaylor BM, Calhoun MT. Microbiology of therapeutic water. *Clin Manage Phys Ther.* 1991;11:34–37.

Knoepfli I, Pederson T. An effective method of sterilizing hydrotherapy equipment. *Phys Ther.* 1962;42:514.

McGuckin MB, Thorpe RJ, Abrutyn E. Hydrotherapy: an outbreak of *Pseudomonas aeruginosa* wound infections related to Hubbard tank treatments. *Arch Phys Med Rehabil.* 1981;62:283–285.

McMillan J, Hargiss C, Nourse A, Williams O. Procedure for decontamination of hydrotherapy equipment. *Phys Ther.* 1976;56:567–570.

Miller JK, LeForest NT, Hedberg M, Chapman V. Surveillance and control of Hubbard tank contaminants. *Phys Ther.* 1970;50:1482–1487.

Nelson RM, Reed JR, Kenton DM. Microbiological evaluation of decontamination procedures for hydrotherapy tanks. *Phys Ther.* 1972;52:919–923.

Page C. The whirlpool bath and cross-infections. *Arch Phys Med Rehabil.* 1954;35:97–98.

Simonetti A, Miller R, Gristina J. Efficacy of povidone-iodine in the disinfection of whirlpool bath and Hubbard tanks. *Phys Ther.* 1972;52:1277–1282.

Sykes JH. Calcium hypochlorite for disinfection of hydrotherapy equipment. *Phys Ther.* 1963;43:345–347.

Shortwave Diathermy

DESCRIPTION

Shortwave diathermy offers heat by the conversion of high-frequency electromagnetic energy to heat energy in patient tissues. The frequency most often
used is 27.12 MHz with a wavelength of 11 m. This frequency, with a narrow
band surrounding it, is one of several frequency bands that have been set aside
for medical use by the Federal Communications Commission (FCC) to eliminate radio interference.

Shortwave diathermy can be delivered as either continuous current or a
pulsed electromagnetic field (PEMF). Pulsed shortwave diathermy is produced
by periodically interrupting the flow of the high-frequency current so that it is
on for a brief period and off for a period equal to or longer than the period the
current flows. The "off" period allows the heat created during the "on" period
to dissipate. If this technique is used at sufficient intensities or for treatment
times that are long enough to produce heat, the effects are the same as the
heating effects of continuous diathermy.

Shortwave diathermy uses either a condenser field or an induction field
to produce heat. The condenser field uses the patient's tissues as the dielectric
between two conducting electrodes. Heat is produced by vibration and distor-
tion of the molecules of the tissues. The heat is strongest where the density of
the field is greatest, which is usually near the electrodes; thus, the heat may be
fairly superficial. Theoretically, if the tissues to be heated constitute a parallel
circuit (i.e., allow alternate pathways for the current), then the good conductors
such as muscles and blood carry the majority of the current and are heated
most. If the tissues form a series circuit, with the current passing through each
tissue in turn, the electrical resistance of the nonconductors such as fat and fi-
brous tissue causes them to be heated as well. The air-spaced plates (Figure
4–1) use a condenser field.

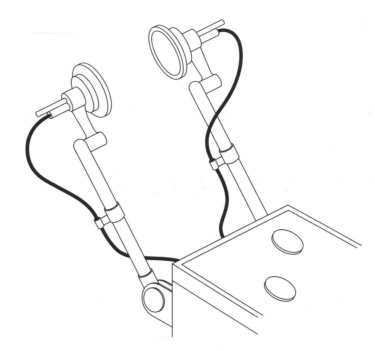

Figure 4–1. Shortwave diathermy equipped with air-spaced plates.

The induction field method places the patient in the electromagnetic field of the electrodes so that current is induced in the conductive tissues of the patient. Heating by this method is primarily in the more superficial muscle layers with the more deeply placed muscles being heated by conduction of heat from overlying ones. Both continuous and pulsed shortwave methods use a drum applicator or monode to produce an induction field (Figure 4–2). Some

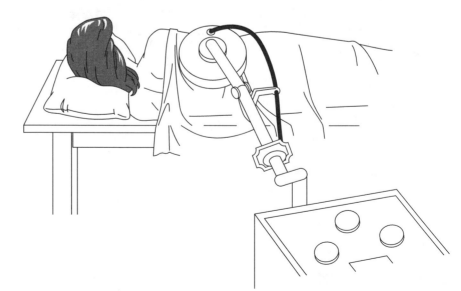

Figure 4–2. Shortwave diathermy equipped with a drum applicator or monode.

units provide two such applicators, which are then called diplodes. In the past, long induction cables (Figure 4–3) were also used for inducing current into tissues, but the method is no longer used.

To summarize, use of a condenser field places the patient in the actual electrical circuit, and the use of an induction field places the patient in the electromagnetic field produced by the equipment. In actuality, there is a great deal of overlap between the two methods. Condenser fields exist even when using inductive techniques, and conductive tissues are heated regardless of which electrode arrangement is used. Thus, there is not as much selective heating of various tissues as once was supposed. Either method is capable of introducing heat to the superficial musculature.[1]

PURPOSE AND EFFECTS

The effects of deep conversive heat are similar to those of other heat sources.

1. Increased metabolism in the tissues in which heat is absorbed.

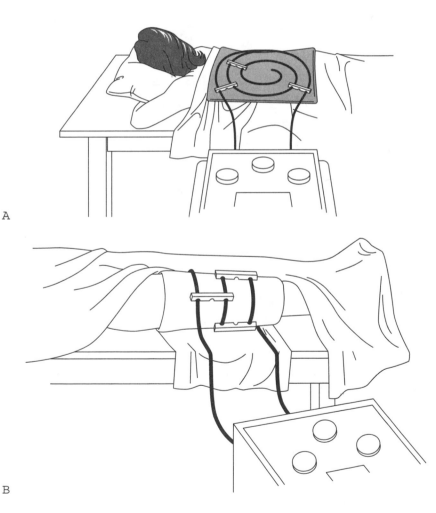

A

B

Figure 4–3. Shortwave diathermy equipped with an induction cable. A. The cable formed into a pancake. B. The cable used as an induction coil.

2. Increased perspiration in the area of absorption.
3. Linear increase in oxygen tension with increased tissue temperature.[2]
4. Local vasodilatation with hyperemia[3,4] in response to increased demands for nutrients or from stimulation of cells that release a histamine-like substance.
5. Muscle relaxation via effects on the muscle spindles and golgi tendon organs.[5]
6. Increased capillary pressure and cell permeability, which can promote local swelling. On the other hand, PEMF has been shown to reduce the edema associated with acute ankle sprains.[6]
7. Increased extensibility of connective tissue in conjunction with stretching exercises.[7–10]
8. Increased body temperature, respiratory and pulse rates, and decreased blood pressure if applied long enough or systemically. These responses of the body act to dissipate the excess heat and maintain a thermal equilibrium.

ADVANTAGE

The primary advantage of using shortwave diathermy as opposed to the radiant or conductive heating methods is the possibility of reaching deeper tissues.

DISADVANTAGES

1. With some of the methods of application, the area being treated is not visible.
2. Because of the electrical origin of the heat, shortwave diathermy is potentially more hazardous than radiant or conductive heat sources.
3. The equipment is costly and time-consuming to set up properly.

INDICATIONS

1. Subacute and chronic inflammatory conditions of superficial joints—use with caution; deep heating may cause collagen destruction within joints with rheumatoid arthritis.[11,12]
2. Subacute and chronic traumatic and inflammatory conditions in muscle.
3. Indirect heating for peripheral vascular disease (i.e., placement on an area of the trunk for increasing blood flow to the extremities without directly heating the extremities).

CONTRAINDICATIONS

1. Acute inflammatory conditions such as sprains and strains may be aggravated by heating.
2. Already existing fever may be elevated further by systemic heating.

3. Malignancies may metastasize due to the increased blood flow produced by heating.[1]
4. Active bleeding such as menses or that which occurs with acute trauma may be prolonged.
5. Patients with cardiac insufficiency may not be able to tolerate the additional stress on the heart produced by generalized heating.
6. Older adults and children less than 4 years old have unreliable thermoregulatory systems and may develop fever quite easily as a result of generalized heat treatments.
7. Patients with peripheral vascular disease have diminished capacity to meet the increased metabolic demands if tissues in the affected extremities are heated directly. Heating a remote area with the intent of producing a reflex vasodilatation in the skin of the affected extremities is an alternative treatment.[13,14]
8. Tissues devitalized by x-ray therapy should not be heated.
9. Any metal in the treatment site that cannot be removed may become hot and damage surrounding tissue.
10. Ischemic tissue may burn due to inadequate blood flow.
11. The electromagnetic energy may interfere with the function of pacemakers, especially demand pacemakers. DO NOT TREAT PATIENTS WEARING PACEMAKERS WITHOUT CONSULTING WITH THE MANUFACTURER OF THE PACEMAKER.
12. Patients who are generally debilitated cannot tolerate strong generalized heating.
13. Shortwave diathermy should not be used over the pregnant uterus, especially during the first trimester, because of the risk of producing bleeding or miscarriage.
14. Infections can spread in the presence of heat.
15. Shortwave diathermy should not be used over the epiphyses of growing bones because of the risk of producing growth disturbances.

PRECAUTIONS

1. Due to the electromagnetic radiation, electronic or magnetic equipment must be removed from the field. The field includes the machine, the electrodes, and the entire length of the wires that connect the electrodes to the unit. This caution also pertains to hearing aids or watches worn by either the patient or the operator.
2. Avoid or correct situations that tend to concentrate the field.
   a. Ischemic areas.
   b. Metal in the treatment area.
   c. Open wounds or moist dressings.
   d. Uneven spacing of the electrodes.
   e. Perspiration.
   f. Uneven pressure of the electrodes.
3. Patients who are poor judges of heat levels should be treated with caution, if at all.
4. Patients with sensory impairment should be treated with caution.
5. Because adipose tissue has such high electrical resistance, obese patients may experience excessive heat superficially.

INSTRUCTIONS

1. Instruct the patient regarding what you are going to do, what benefits to expect, and what you expect of her.
2. Have the patient remove all clothing and metal in the area to be treated. Inspect the skin for integrity and temperature sensation. Moisture and metal in the field can concentrate the current and potentially cause burns. Clothing on the part to be treated prevents the practitioner from drying the skin as perspiration develops. Additionally, some synthetic fabrics (e.g., nylon) can cause excessive heating by trapping moisture.
3. Position the patient on a plinth or chair in an appropriate, comfortable, and secure position, and drape her. Wooden plinths or chairs are required because they cannot conduct the current. Avoid foam rubber pillows, which can absorb moisture and overheat.
4. Explain to the patient that she should not move around once the treatment has started. Except with PEMF, the patient should feel only a mild sensation of warmth. Patients experience no heat sensation when PEMF is used. Provide a call system should the patient require assistance later during the treatment.
5. Select a treatment method and set it up according to the following instructions. Selection depends on the structures to be heated and the patient position.
   a. Condenser field—air-spaced plates. The plates are metal electrodes encased in a plastic or glass housing, with or without spacers. Position these plates over the area to the treated, considering the following points.
      (1) Spacing.
         (a) The plates should be about 1 to 3 in. (2.5 to 7.5 cm) from the patient to make the field even. If electrodes are much closer, heat will be superficial, because the field is more dense near them. Wider spacing allows a more even field and deeper heating. If electrodes are much farther from the skin, the unit may not function (Figure 4–4A and C).
         (b) Wider spacing is indicated for uneven surfaces so that the field does not concentrate over bony prominences. Spacing is measured from the highest part of the skin surface to be treated.
         (c) Spacing should be equal under both electrodes. If it is not, more heat is produced under the electrode that is closer to the skin (Figure 4–4B).
         (d) If spacing rings are present, they should be placed so that air can circulate beneath them; they should not contact the skin.
         (e) Air-spacing is best to allow for air circulation, but dry terry cloth toweling may be placed on the part to absorb and dissipate perspiration as it forms.
      (2) Position.
         (a) Determine the tissues to be treated and position the electrodes so that they provide heat to the desired tissues. Non-

conductive tissues should be treated by the contraplanar method (i.e., placing the electrodes on opposite sides of the part). Conductive tissues should be treated with a longitudinal or coplanar approach so that the electrodes are on the same surface of the part.

(b) The electrodes should be parallel to the skin surface or the field will be concentrated where they are closer to the skin (Figure 4–4D).

(c) The adjacent edges of the electrodes should be farther from each other than the total spacing between the electrodes and the skin (Figure 4–4E).

b. Induction field method—monode.

(1) The monode contains a coil of wire that is prespaced within a plastic housing. This permits application using air-spacing, a single layer of toweling, or a thick layer of blanketing (Figure 4–5).

(2) Although air-spacing is usually most desirable, padding may be used over uneven surfaces.

6. Take care that the cables from the electrodes do not cross each other, touch each other, or touch the patient.

7. Whenever possible, try to position the unit in such a way that the patient cannot handle it, the electrodes, or the wires.

8. Be sure the electrode cables are plugged into the appropriate terminals on the unit.

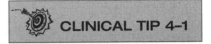

CLINICAL TIP 4–1

Treating Areas With Skin Contact Using Shortwave Diathermy

Areas in which the skin of one body part can contact the skin of another part should be separated with absorptive padding. For example, if the anterior or posterior aspect of the shoulder is treated, a rolled towel should be placed in the axilla to absorb perspiration and prevent the arm and trunk from contacting each other.

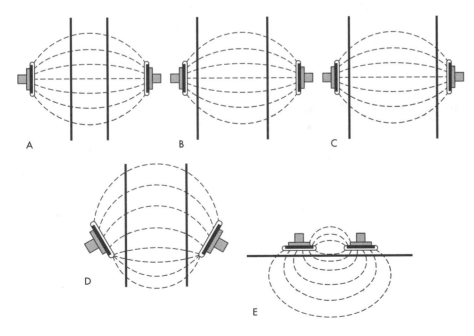

Figure 4–4. Electrode spacing with air-spaced plates. The solid lines represent the surface of the skin. A. The electrodes are properly spaced, creating even, deep heat. B. The electrodes are unevenly spaced, creating more heat under the left one. C. The electrodes are too close to the skin, concentrating the field and creating superficial heat. D. The plates are not parallel to the skin, creating hot spots where they are closer. E. The electrodes are too close to each other, concentrating the field between them and potentially creating a hot spot.

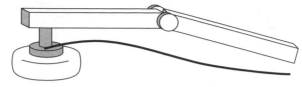

Figure 4–5. Drum electrode or monode.

9. Once the treatment method has been selected, the patient should keep movement to a minimum. Explain to the patient that motion within the field changes the spacing and, thus, the heat distribution.

10. Turn on the machine and allow any warm-up time that may be necessary.

11. Most units tune automatically. If so, after it is tuned, adjust the intensity to a level that produces a mild warmth.

12. Older units require manual tuning. To tune manually, turn the output dial to about one third of the total output. Then adjust the tuning dial to tune the patient circuit to resonance with the oscillator circuit. As the tuning dial is turned, the needle in the meter rises and falls. When the needle indicates its highest reading, the circuits are tuned. Set the tuning dial to maintain the highest reading.

13. Check the patient frequently. Attend to any complaints of discomfort from the positioning or excessive heat at once. Be sure the unit remains in tune.

14. At the conclusion of treatment, return all dials to the zero position, remove all apparatus, cover the patient, and allow her to rest for about 10 minutes.

15. Perform all indicated posttreatment evaluation procedures, including checking physiologic status and skin condition.

16. Document patient position, method used, spacing and position of the electrodes, and patient response.

RESPONSES TO TREATMENT AND TREATMENT MODIFICATION

A normal response includes pink skin and perspiration. If the patient has very dark skin, changes in skin color may not be observed. If the skin is red or the patient reports excessive heat, adjust the spacing of the electrodes. Be certain that perspiration is not accumulating. If the patient develops very red skin or blisters, remove the apparatus immediately and place a cold or ice pack on the area. File an incident report.

DOSAGE

Intensity

The heat produced by shortwave diathermy should be very gentle, because much of it is produced deep to the superficially located heat receptors.

Duration

The duration of treatment is usually 20 to 30 minutes. Subacute inflammatory conditions may be treated for 10 to 15 minutes.

Frequency

Shortwave diathermy may be given daily or twice daily for subacute conditions and less often for chronic conditions.

HOME USE

Because of the inherent hazard concerning its use, the cost of the equipment, and the lack of availability of portable equipment, shortwave diathermy is not appropriate for home use.

REFERENCES

1. Lehmann JF, DeLateur BJ. Therapeutic heat. In: Lehmann JF, ed. *Therapeutic Heat and Cold.* 3rd ed. Baltimore: Williams & Wilkins; 1982.
2. Rabkin JM, Hunt TK. Local heat increases blood flow and oxygen tension in wounds. *Arch Surg.* 1987;122:221–225.
3. Lehmann JF, Silverman DR, Baum BA, et al. Temperature distributions in the human thigh, produced by infrared, hot pack and microwave applications. *Arch Phys Med Rehabil.* 1966;47:291–299.
4. McMeeken J. Tissue temperature and blood flow: a research based overview of electrophysical modalities. *Aust J Physiother.* 1994;40(4):49–57.
5. Mense S. Effects of temperature on the discharges of muscle spindles and tendon organs. *Pflügers Arch.* 1978;374:159–166.
6. Pennington GM, Danley DL, Sumko MH, Bucknell A, Nelson JH. Pulsed, non-thermal, high-frequency electromagnetic energy (Diapulse) in the treatment of grade I and grade II ankle sprains. *Milit Med.* 1993;158:101–104.
7. Lehmann JF, Masock AJ, Warren CG, Koblanski JN. Effect of therapeutic temperatures on tendon extensibility. *Arch Phys Med Rehabil.* 1970;51:481–487.
8. Lentell G, Hetherington T, Eagan J, Morgan M. The use of thermal agents to influence the effectiveness of a low-load prolonged stretch. *J Orthop Sports Phys Ther.* 1992;16:200–207.
9. Prentice WE. An electromyographic analysis of the effectiveness of heat or cold and stretching for inducing relaxation in injured muscle. *J Orthop Sports Phys Ther.* 1982;3:133–140.
10. Warren CG, Lehmann JF, Koblanski JN. Heat and stretch procedures: an evaluation using rat tail tendon. *Arch Phys Med Rehabil.* 1976;57:122–126.
11. Harris ED, McCroskery PA. The influence of temperature and fibril stability on degradation of cartilage collagen by rheumatoid synovial collagenase. *N Engl J Med.* 1974;290:1–6.
12. Feibel A, Fast A. Deep heating of joints: a reconsideration. *Arch Phys Med Rehabil.* 1976;57:613.
13. Abramson DI, Tuck S, Chu LSW, et al. Indirect vasodilatation in thermotherapy. *Arch Phys Med Rehabil.* 1965;46:412–420.
14. Wessman HC, Kottke FJ. The effect of indirect heating on peripheral blood flow, pulse rate, blood pressure, and temperature. *Arch Phys Med Rehabil.* 1967;48:567–576.

ADDITIONAL READINGS

Amundson H. Thermotherapy and cryotherapy—effects on joint degeneration in rheumatoid arthritis. *Physiother Can.* 1979;31:258–262.

Barker AT, Barlow PS, Porter J, et al. A double-blind clinical trial of low power pulsed shortwave therapy in the treatment of a soft tissue injury. *Physiotherapy.* 1985;71: 500–504.

Barnett M. Shortwave diathermy for herpes zoster. *Physiotherapy.* 1979;61:217.

Benson TB, Copp EP. The effects of therapeutic forms of heat and ice on the pain threshold of the normal shoulder. *Rheumatol Rehabil.* 1974;13:101–104.

Brown M, Baker RD. Effect of pulsed short wave diathermy on skeletal muscle injury in rabbits. *Phys Ther.* 1987;67:208–214.

Chastain P. The effect of deep heat on isometric strength. *Phys Ther.* 1978;58:543–546.

Clarke GR, Willis LA, Stenner L, Nichols PJR. Evaluation of physiotherapy in the treatment of osteoarthrosis of the knee. *Rheumatol Rehabil.* 1974;13:190–197.

Dillon J, Herbert R. A retrospective study of the effects of short wave on the birth outcomes of physiotherapists. *Aust J Physiother.* 1985;31:33.

Hamilton DE, Bywaters EGL, Please NW. A controlled trial of various forms of physiotherapy in arthritis. *Br Med J.* 1959;1:542–544.

Harris R. Effect of short wave diathermy on radio-sodium clearance from the knee joint in the normal and in rheumatoid arthritis. *Arch Phys Med Rehabil.* 1960;42:241–249.

Harris R, Millard JB. Clearance of radioactive sodium from the knee joint. *Clin Sci.* 1956;15:9–15.

Hayne CR. Pulsed high frequency energy—its place in physiotherapy. *Physiotherapy.* 1984;70:459–466.

Heath J. The effects of shortwave diathermy, microwave and ultrasonics on demand pacemakers and ventrical inhibited pacemakers. *Aust J Physiother.* 1974;20:144–145.

Hollander JL, Horvath SM. The influence of physical therapy procedures on the intra-articular temperature of normal and arthritic subjects. *Am J Med Sci.* 1949;218:543–548.

Hovind H, Nielson SL. Local blood flow after short wave diathermy: preliminary report. *Arch Phys Med Rehabil.* 1974;55:217–221.

Jan M, Lai J. The effects of physiotherapy on osteoarthritic knees of females. *J Formosan Med Assn.* 1991;90:1008–1013.

Kloth L, Morrison MA, Ferguson BH. *Therapeutic Microwave and Shortwave Diathermy: A Review of Thermal Effectiveness, Safe Use, and State of the Art: 1984.* Rockville, Md: US Department of Health and Human Services; 1984. Publication FDA 85-8237.

Lehmann J, DeLateur BJ, Stonebridge JB. Selective muscle heating by shortwave diathermy with a helical coil. *Arch Phys Med Rehabil.* 1969;50:117–123.

Lehmann JF, McDougall JA, Grey AW, et al. Heating patterns produced by shortwave diathermy applicators in tissue substitute models. *Arch Phys Med Rehabil.* 1983; 64:575–577.

Lehmann JF, McMillan JA, Brunner GD, Blumberg JB. Comparative study of the efficiency of short-wave, microwave and ultrasonic diathermy in heating the hip joint. *Arch Phys Med Rehabil.* 1959;40:510–512.

McCray RE, Patton NJ. Pain relief of trigger points: a comparison of moist heat and shortwave diathermy. *J Orthop Sports Phys Ther.* 1984;5:175–178.

Morrissey L. Effect of pulsed short-wave diathermy upon volume blood flow through the calf of the leg. *Phys Ther.* 1966;46:946–952.

Oliver DE. Pulsed electro-magnetic energy—what is it? *Physiotherapy.* 1984;70:458–459.

Quirk AS, Newman RJ, Newman KJ. An evaluation of interferential therapy, shortwave diathermy and exercise in the treatment of osteoarthrosis of the knee. *Physiotherapy.* 1985;71:55–57.

Salmon J. Physiotherapy in intramuscular lesions. *Aust J Physiother.* 1973;18:18–22.

Santiesteban AJ. The role of physical agents in the treatment of spine pain. *Clin Orthop.* 1983;179:24–30.

Silverman DR, Pendleton L. A comparison of the effects of continuous and pulsed shortwave diathermy on peripheral circulation. *Arch Phys Med Rehabil.* 1968;49:429–436.

Strangel L. The value of cryotherapy and thermotherapy in the relief of pain. *Physiother Can.* 1975;27:135–139.

Svarcová J, Trnavsky K, Zvárová J. The influence of ultrasound, galvanic currents and shortwave diathermy on pain intensity in patients with osteoarthritis. *Scand J Rheumatol.* 1988; 67(suppl):83–85.

Trock DJ, Bollet AJ, Markoll R. The effect of pulsed electromagnetic fields in the treatment of osteoarthritis of the knee and cervical spine. Report of randomized, double blind, placebo controlled trials. *J Rheumatol.* 1994;21:1903–1911.

Vanharanta H. Effect of short-wave diathermy on mobility and radiological stage of the knee in the development of experimental osteoarthritis. *Am J Phys Med.* 1982;61:59–65.

Vanharanta H, Eronen I, Videman T. Shortwave diathermy effects on ^{35}S-sulfate uptake and glycosaminoglycan concentration in rabbit knee tissue. *Arch Phys Med Rehabil.* 1982;63:25–28.

Verrier M, Falconer K, Crawford JS. Comparison of tissue temperature following two shortwave diathermy techniques. *Physiother Can.* 1977;61:21–25.

Wagstaff P, Wagstaff S, Downey M. A pilot study to compare the efficacy of continuous and pulsed magnetic energy [short-wave diathermy] on the relief of low back pain. *Physiotherapy.* 1986;72:563–566.

Webber BA. Interference to cardiac pacemakers. *Physiother Can.* 1975;61:276.

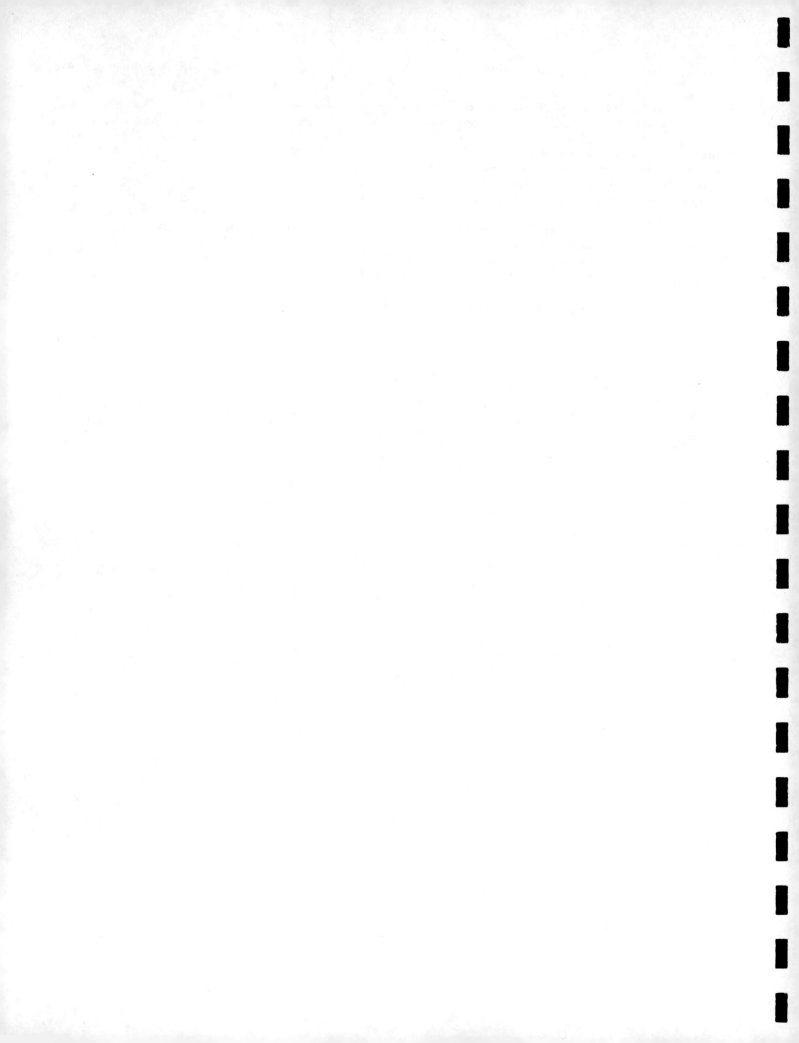

Ultrasound

DESCRIPTION

Ultrasound is a name given to sound waves that are of such high frequency that they are not detectable by the human ear. The frequency for medical ultrasound in the United States is 800,000 to 3,000,000 Hz (0.8 to 3 MHz). Ultrasound waves are produced by means of a piezoelectric crystal. When an alternating current is impressed on this crystal, distortions of its molecular structure occur, and it vibrates, producing mechanical waves identical to sound waves. The frequency of the waves is determined by the size of the crystal and the frequency of the impressed current. These waves require an elastic medium through which to travel. As they travel, they alternately compress (condensation phase) and release (rarefaction phase) the molecules of the medium, imparting energy to them. The energy from the waves may produce thermal or mechanical effects where they are absorbed.

Ultrasound energy can be delivered continuously or pulsed. The theory behind pulsed ultrasound is that the energy is delivered in packets or bursts with a rest time ("off" time) between packets. During the "off" time, any heat that was created as a result of the period of energy transmission dissipates. Thus, pulsed ultrasound minimizes heat production and allows for the use of any nonthermal or mechanical effects imparted by the energy. The time during which the energy is being delivered (the "on" time) is related to the total of the "on" and "off" times and expressed as a duty cycle. Most equipment offers 20% and 50% duty cycles. The product of the duty cycle and the intensity suggests the comparable intensity of continuous ultrasound. For example, if pulsed ultrasound were delivered at a temporal peak intensity of 1.0 W/cm^2 and a 20% duty cycle, the energy would be comparable to that delivered by continuous ultrasound at 0.2 W/cm^2 (temporal average intensity). At present, the evidence of the effectiveness of pulsed ultrasound is equivocal.[1-3]

PURPOSE AND EFFECTS

Sound waves are capable of reflection, refraction, penetration, and absorption. When applied to human tissue, they are absorbed by various tissues with the production of heat. Absorption is greatest in tissues with a high proportion of protein and in dense tissues. Penetration is greatest of all heat modalities, with significant heating 2 in. (5 cm) below the surface.[4,5] Because of reflection, heat is greatest at tissue interfaces, especially those of widely different acoustic impedance. For example, because of the mismatch in acoustic impedance, ultrasound is capable of producing significant heating in the synovial tissues and capsule in front of the bone.[6] For the same reason, much heat is produced at the periosteum. There is very little temperature increase in adipose tissue.[7]

Nearly all of the ultrasound waves are reflected by air; therefore, ultrasound requires direct contact in the form of a coupling medium to facilitate transfer of energy to the tissue. The coupling medium fills incongruities between the transducer faceplate and the skin.

In addition to the familiar effects produced by a rise in temperature (see those listed for shortwave diathermy), there is evidence of nonthermal effects resulting from vibration of the molecules.[8]

1. Separation of collagen fibers with a resultant increase in the extensibility of connective tissue such as in joint capsule, ligament, tendon, adhesions, and scars.[9] Although mechanical effects play a role in the greater extensibility, the increase is mostly due to the thermal effects.[10]
2. Increased membrane permeability allowing for increased ionic exchange.[11]

ADVANTAGES

1. Ultrasound is capable of producing significant temperature changes deep within the tissue.
2. It is a very local treatment with few generalized responses.
3. Application times are usually short.

DISADVANTAGES

1. Very little sensation is associated with treatment, making dosage difficult to monitor.
2. Pressure is exerted on the part to be treated, aggravating any tenderness.
3. Because ultrasound waves are highly focused upon leaving the transducer, only small areas can be treated at one time. Ultrasound is not appropriate for large body surfaces.

INDICATIONS

1. Soft tissue shortening (joint contractures, scarring).
2. Subacute and chronic inflammation.
3. Painful conditions such as muscle guarding, neuroma, or trigger areas.

4. Warts.[12]
5. Wound healing.[13,14]

CONTRAINDICATIOINS

1. Arterial circulation must be sufficient to meet the increased metabolic demand.
2. Increased blood flow could enhance any local bleeding already present.
3. Ultrasound over the eyes could cause cavitation in the fluid compartments.
4. Sonating over a gravid uterus could cause cavitation in the amniotic fluid and potential damage to the fetus.
5. Cancer may metastasize due to the increased blood flow.[15]
6. Do not sonate over the spinal cord after a laminectomy; cavitation can occur in the cerebrospinal fluid.
7. Infectious processes can be accelerated by heat.
8. Do not sonate over the carotid sinus or cervical ganglia. Doing so could cause disturbance of the normal pacing of the heart or stimulate baroreceptors.
9. Intracapsular heating may promote accelerated destruction of articular cartilage in acute inflammatory joint pathologies.[16]

PRECAUTIONS

1. Care should be taken to maintain consistent energy transfer, or burns could result.
   a. Keep the transducer moving.
   b. Maintain even contact.
   c. Remove air bubbles.
2. Keep off bony prominences to eliminate the possibility of concentrating energy at the periosteum.
3. Do not hold the transducer in the air for longer than a few seconds. Air does not transmit the waves, and the crystal could shatter or depolarize, its cement could melt, or the transducer could become very hot. Some generators have a feedback system that prevents the crystal from overheating.
4. Avoid the use of intensities higher than those considered therapeutic. High intensities produce cavitation, which is a phenomenon whereby bubbles of dissolved gas form and grow during each rarefaction phase. Through their vibration and absorption of energy, they can create sites of energy concentration or actually tear tissue.
5. Be cautious about sonating over anesthetized skin, because the patient must rely on thermal feedback to report excessive heating.

INSTRUCTIONS

1. Instruct the patient about the treatment and what is expected.
2. Position and drape the patient for comfort, modesty, and easy accessibility, keeping the part to be treated uncovered. Position the equipment to allow for comfortable use of both hands.

3. Check the equipment and patient sensation. Tell the patient to expect to feel the transducer moving over the skin and that any sensation of warmth should be extremely mild. Any other sensation should be reported immediately.

4. Identify the area to be treated. Because the waves are so local, they must be directed specifically at the site of pathology, and the area must be small. A good rule of thumb for determining the size of the area of treatment is to treat an area no larger than two to three times the size of the effective radiating area (ERA).[4] The ERA refers to the amount of the transducer faceplate that actually produces sound waves and usually relates to the size of the crystal. In some units, the faceplate is larger than the ERA. If an area that is more than two to three times the size of the ERA is treated, the energy is distributed too broadly, and therapeutic temperature in the target tissue is not reached.

5. Gaining access to the site may involve positioning the part in such a way as to move the target tissue out from under overlying tissue.

6. If available on the generator, select an appropriate frequency range. Sound waves at 1 MHz diverge more as they leave the transducer but penetrate deeply (1 to 2 in. [2.5 to 5 cm]). High-frequency (3 MHz) waves are absorbed more easily, raise temperatures more quickly, and do not penetrate as deeply (0.4 to 1 in. [1 to 2.5 cm]).[4] Consequently, waves of 3 MHz are more appropriate for shallower targets.

7. Because sound waves of ultrasonic frequencies do not travel through air, a coupling medium is necessary. This medium should have the following characteristics:
   a. It must transmit waves readily rather than absorb them. Oil absorbs ultrasound waves and produces superficial heat.[7]
   b. It must be inert; that is, it should not transfer molecules into the patient's tissues (see phonophoresis).
   c. It must allow good contact throughout the entire treatment; that is, it should not liquefy and flow from the area.
   d. It must contain no dissolved gases that would reflect the waves and prevent transmission.

8. Two methods of coupling, using different media, are available.
   a. Conductive gel or glycerol contact coupling. Apply to clean skin enough conductive gel or glycerol to last throughout the treatment. Apply the transducer faceplate directly to the coupling medium, with firm, but not heavy, contact that must be maintained throughout the treatment. Make sure there are no air gaps. This method works best with smooth surfaces.
   b. Water coupling. For irregular surfaces, the part to be treated may be immersed in tepid water. Degassed water is preferable. The water may be boiled and cooled or allowed to stand for a while so that air bubbles do not settle on the patient and cause spotty energy distribution. Hold the transducer faceplate 0.5 to 1.0 in. (1.25 to 2.5 cm) away from the surface of the skin and parallel to it. Subaqueous treatment is of dubious effectiveness because therapeutic temperatures are not reached, especially if the water is not degassed.[4,17]

   Heating is best with 1-MHz ultrasound, especially if a metal rather than plastic container is used.[18] Without compensations in dosage, subaqueous ultrasound does not increase tissue temperature

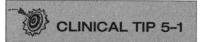

CLINICAL TIP 5-1

Focusing the Sound Waves to the Target Tissue

Because the sound waves leave the transducer in a columnar form, they must be focused on the specific tissue. For example, if you wish to sonate the supraspinatus tendon, position the patient in shoulder extension, internal rotation, and adduction to bring the tendon out from under the acromion.

as much as contact ultrasound, and any temperature increases are diminished as the distance from the transducer faceplate to the skin increases.[5] When delivering treatments under water, an additional 0.5 W/cm^2 may be used to compensate for absorption by the water.

9. To ensure safety with either type of coupling, keep the transducer moving when applying the sound waves to the patient. This practice prevents energy concentration in one area and thus the possibility of burning. Use circular movements, establishing a rhythmic pattern at a rate of about 1.6 in. (4 cm) per second. Each circle should cover about one half the area of the previous circle. Be careful not to linger over any single area. A moving transducer is necessary to prevent hot spots due to the lack of uniformity of the field. The beam nonuniformity ratio (BNR), a measure of the uniformity of the ultrasound beam, refers to the relationship between the peak amplitude of the waves in the field and the average amplitude. The lower the BNR, the more uniform the field. With a low BNR (e.g., 2:1) movement of the transducer can be slower than with a high BNR (e.g., 5:1). To minimize the effects of refraction and allow for deepest penetration, the transducer should be held parallel to the skin.

10. Establish the appropriate dosage. Dosage is governed by power and time. For continuous ultrasound, power or spatial average intensity is measured in watts per square centimeter of the surface of the crystal or the ERA. Set the intensity while moving the transducer on the body surface. Be sure to maintain the movement if further adjustments of dosage must be made.

11. In any condition, once judgment of a target dose has been made, the patient's subjective tolerance is the ultimate determinant.

12. At the conclusion of the treatment, be sure the power is off before removing the transducer. Clean or dry the patient. Clean the transducer before returning it to its receptacle.

13. Perform all appropriate posttreatment evaluations, including skin inspection and checking general physiologic responses.

14. Document the mode, duty cycle if applicable, intensity, duration, frequency, and all patient responses.

RESPONSES TO TREATMENT AND TREATMENT MODIFICATION

The patient should experience nothing but the gentlest warmth. If the patient complains of sharp pain, especially over bony prominences, the periosteum may be receiving too much energy. Because the periosteum is the tissue immediately in front of bone, the acoustic mismatch causes a great deal of reflection to the periosteum. The lack of soft tissue coverage makes bony prominences at risk for periosteal burning. If the patient expresses such a complaint, decrease the intensity immediately.

DOSAGE

Intensity

The safe range of intensity for a moving transducer is 0.5 to 3 W/cm^2. Using 1 MHz continuous ultrasound, doses of 0.5 W/cm^2 have been shown to be incapable of increasing tissue temperature to the therapeutic range.[4] Goal of treat-

> **CLINICAL TIP 5-2**
>
> **Effect of Ultrasound on Nerve Conduction Velocity**
>
> Sonation can affect motor nerve conduction velocity, depending on the dosage.[19] Low intensities (0.5 W/cm²) and high intensities (3 W/cm²) have been shown to cause velocity to increase, whereas moderate intensities (1 to 2 W/cm²) caused the velocity to decrease. Ultrasound has been shown to increase sensory nerve conduction velocity.[20-23]

ment and acuteness of the condition must be considered when establishing power. Connective tissue shortening should be treated with high dosages to maximize temperature increase. Painful conditions may respond better to more moderate doses. The more acute the condition, the lower the dose should be, thus reserving stronger doses for chronic problems.

Duration

Duration of treatment is usually short, 5 to 10 minutes per site.[11,24] Less than 3 minutes of treatment is ineffective for achieving any physiologic response. Using 1-MHz frequency, therapeutic temperature is not reached before 10 minutes of treatment.[4] Using a 3-MHz frequency causes tissue temperature to increase faster.[4] Chronic, deep-seated problems may require longer doses. Initial treatments may be shorter than subsequent ones.

Frequency

Initially, treatment may be given daily and then decreased with improvement of the patient's condition.

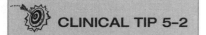

Phonophoresis

DESCRIPTION

Phonophoresis is a process in which whole medicinal molecules are driven across the skin and into the subcutaneous tissue by means of ultrasound.[25,26]

PURPOSE AND EFFECTS

The major purpose of using phonophoresis is to introduce medicinal molecules to a local area without invasion of the skin. Thus, it is a painless and safer means of treatment than injection of the same substance. Both thermal and nonthermal effects may account for the ability of ultrasound to facilitate introduction of medicinal molecules across the skin. Increase in the kinetic energy of the molecules is a thermal effect, and increase in cell membrane permeability is both thermal and nonthermal.[11] Once introduced, the medication has the same effects as it would if introduced by injection.

In some states, certain practitioners are not permitted by law to dispense medications, so the patient may need a prescription from a physician to obtain the preparation and bring it to the practitioner for treatment.

INDICATIONS

The most common uses are for subcutaneous inflammatory and painful conditions using anesthetics (e.g., lidocaine) or nonsteroidal[27] or steroidal[28,29] anti-inflammatory drugs (e.g., salicylate, hydrocortisone, dexamethasone). Dexamethasone appears to transmit ultrasound better than hydrocortisone.[30] When using hydrocortisone, a concentration of about 10% appears to be more effective than one of 1%.[29] The deposition of the steroidal medications is not as deep as the penetration of the ultrasound waves, and there is little evidence that medication reaches muscle or tendon.[30]

CONTRAINDICATIONS AND PRECAUTIONS

1. Because ultrasound is used for phonophoresis, the contraindications and precautions listed for ultrasound also apply.
2. Check a *Physician's Desk Reference*[31] for any conditions that are contraindicated for the drug.

INSTRUCTIONS

1. Prepare the patient in the same manner as for treatment with ultrasound alone.
2. The medication and carrier are often applied to the skin as the coupling medium. The effectiveness of phonophoresis depends in part on the transmissivity of the carrier. If the carrier does not transmit ultrasound, it cannot deposit medication. To test whether the carrier and medication can transmit adequately, use gummed tape around the transducer, and form a well about 0.4 in. (1 cm) deep. Place a layer of the medium on the transducer surface, and fill the well with water. Set the ultrasound unit to 1 to 2 W/cm^2 and increase the intensity. If the medium transmits, the water will be disturbed.[32]

   In general, thick, white creams and gels into which powders have been mixed do not transmit ultrasound.[32,33] In preparing the medication, avoid whipping the medication into the carrier, because trapped air can decrease transmission of the ultrasound by up to 50%.[34]
3. The technique of delivery is the same as for ultrasound alone.
4. Dosage is dependent on the same factors as ultrasound. Do not exceed a safe ultrasound dosage.
5. At the end of the treatment, turn off the equipment, and clean and dry the patient.
6. Perform all appropriate posttreatment evaluations, including a skin inspection and check of general physiologic responses. Be especially alert to systemic responses to the medication.
7. Document the mode of treatment; duty cycle, if applicable; intensity; duration; frequency; medication used; preparation of the medication, including the carrier and dosage; and all patient responses.

RESPONSES TO TREATMENT AND TREATMENT MODIFICATION

As with ultrasound without medication, the patient should experience nothing but the gentlest warmth. If the patient complains of sharp pain, especially over bony prominences, the periosteum may be receiving too much energy. Because the periosteum is the tissue immediately in front of bone, the acoustic mismatch causes a great deal of reflection to the periosteum. The lack of soft tissue coverage makes bony prominences at risk for periosteal burning. If the patient expresses such a complaint, decrease the intensity immediately.

In addition to the responses to the ultrasound treatment, the patient should exhibit the agent-specific response to the medication. Maximum local effects should occur within about 2 hours.[35]

DOSAGE

Intensity

To use the thermal effects of ultrasound, intensities over 1.5 W/cm² are necessary.[24] On the other hand, low-intensity, long-duration doses have been shown to be more effective at transferring medication than high-intensity, short-duration doses.[36] Regardless of the intensity, it is difficult to measure the actual amount of medication introduced.

Duration

Five to 10 minutes of sonation are necessary to reach therapeutic temperatures at 1.0 to 1.5 W/cm² in people with less than 3.2 in. (8 cm) of soft tissue thickness.[24] Sometimes intensities this high can produce discomfort or pain. To counter these effects, low-dose, long-duration treatments of comparable intensity–duration product have been used effectively to transfer medication. For example, 1 W/cm² for 5 minutes theoretically delivers the same ultrasonic energy as 0.3 W/cm² for 17 minutes, although the two doses do not deliver the same amount of medication.[36]

Frequency

The frequency of treatment should be established in consultation with the treating physician to maintain the drug level properly.

REFERENCES

1. Dyson M, Pond JB. The effect of pulsed ultrasound on tissue regeneration. *Physiotherapy.* 1970;56:136–142.
2. Nykänen M. Pulsed ultrasound treatment of the painful shoulder: a randomized, double-blind, placebo-controlled study. *Scand J Rehabil Med.* 1995;27:105–108.
3. Ter Riet G, Kessels AGH, Knipschild P. A randomized clinical trial of ultrasound in the treatment of pressure ulcers. *Phys Ther.* 1996;76:1301–1312.
4. Draper DO, Castel JC, Castel D. Rate of temperature increase in human muscle during 1 MHz and 3 MHz continuous ultrasound. *J Orthop Sports Phys Ther.* 1995;22:142–150.
5. Robertson VJ, Ward AR. Limited interchangeability of methods of applying 1 MHz ultrasound. *Arch Phys Med Rehabil.* 1996;77:379–384.
6. Lehmann JF, DeLateur BJ, Warren CG, Stonebridge JS. Heating produced by ultrasound in bone and soft tissue. *Arch Phys Med Rehabil.* 1967;48:397–401.
7. Ward AR. *Electricity Fields and Waves in Therapy.* Marrickville, NSW, Australia: Science Press; 1986.
8. Lehmann JF, DeLateur BJ. Therapeutic heat. In: Lehmann JF, ed. *Therapeutic Heat and Cold.* 3rd ed. Baltimore: Williams & Wilkins; 1982.
9. Griffin JE. Physiological effects of ultrasound energy as it is used clinically. *Phys Ther.* 1966;46:18–26.
10. Gersten JW. Effect of ultrasound on tendon extensibility. *Am J Phys Med.* 1955;34:362–369.

11. Dyson M. Mechanisms involved in therapeutic ultrasound. *Physiotherapy*. 1987;73: 116–120.
12. Kent H. Plantar wart treatment with ultrasound. *Arch Phys Med Rehabil*. 1959;40:15–18.
13. Byl NN, McKenzie A, Wong T, et al. Incisional wound healing: a controlled study of low and high dose ultrasound. *J Orthop Sports Phys Ther*. 1993;18: 619–628.
14. Dyson M, Suckling J. Stimulation of tissue repair by ultrasound: a survey of the mechanisms involved. *Physiotherapy*. 1978;64:105–108.
15. Sicard-Rosenbaum L, Danoff JV, Guthrie JA, Eckhaus MA. Effects of energy-matched pulsed and continuous ultrasound on tumor growth in mice. *Phys Ther*. 1998;78: 271–277.
16. Harris ED, McCroskery PA. The influence of temperature and fibril stability on degradation of cartilage collagen by rheumatoid synovial collagenase. *N Engl J Med*. 1974; 290:1–6.
17. Forrest G, Rosen K. Ultrasound: effectiveness of ultrasound given under water. *Arch Phys Med Rehabil*. 1989;70:28–29.
18. Robertson VJ, Ward AR. Subaqueous ultrasound: 45kHz and 1MHz machines compared. *Arch Phys Med Rehabil*. 1995;76:569–575.
19. Farmer WC. Effect of intensity of ultrasound on conduction of motor axons. *Phys Ther*. 1968;48:1233–1237.
20. Currier DP, Greathouse D, Swift T. Sensory nerve conduction: effect of ultrasound. *Arch Phys Med Rehabil*. 1978;59:181–185.
21. Currier DP, Kramer JF. Sensory nerve conduction: heating effects of ultrasound and infrared. *Physiother Can*. 1982;34:241–246.
22. Halle JS, Scoville CR, Greathouse DG. Ultrasound's effects on the conduction latency of the superficial radial nerve in man. *Phys Ther*. 1981;61:345–350.
23. Kramer JF. Ultrasound: evaluation of its mechanical and thermal effects. *Arch Phys Med Rehabil*. 1984;65:223–227.
24. Lehmann JF, DeLateur BJ, Stonebridge JB, Warren CG. Therapeutic temperature distribution produced by ultrasound as modified by dosage and volume of tissue exposed. *Arch Phys Med Rehabil*. 1967;48:662–666.
25. Griffin JE, Touchstone JC. Ultrasonic movement of cortisol into pig tissues: I. Movement into paravertebral muscle. *Am J Phys Med*. 1963;42:77–85.
26. Griffin JE, Touchstone JC, Liu AC-Y. Ultrasonic movement of cortisol into pig tissue: II. Movement into paravertebral nerve. *Am J Phys Med*. 1965;44:20–25.
27. Ciccone CD, Leggin BG, Callamaro JJ. Effects of ultrasound and trolamine salicylate phonophoresis on delayed onset muscle soreness. *Phys Ther*. 1991;71:666–678.
28. Griffin JE, Echternach JL, Price RE, Touchstone JC. Patients treated with ultrasonic driven hydrocortisone and with ultrasound alone. *Phys Ther*. 1967;47:594–601.
29. Kleinkort JA, Wood F. Phonophoresis with 1 percent versus 10 percent hydrocortisone. *Phys Ther*. 1975;55:1320–1324.
30. Byl NN, McKenzie A, Halliday B, et al. The effects of phonophoresis with corticosteroids: a controlled pilot study. *J Orthop Sports Phys Ther*. 1993;18:590–600.
31. *Physician's Desk Reference*. 52nd ed. Oradell, NJ: Medical Economics Company; 1998.
32. Cameron MH, Monroe LG. Relative transmission of ultrasound by media customarily used for phonophoresis. *Phys Ther*. 1992;72:142–148.
33. Benson HAE, McElnay JC. Topical non-steroidal anti-inflammatory products as ultrasound couplants: their potential in phonophoresis. *Physiotherapy*. 1994;80:74–76.
34. Warren CG, Koblanski JN, Sigelman RA. Ultrasound coupling media: their relative transmissivity. *Arch Phys Med Rehabil*. 1976;57:218–222.
35. Byl NN. The use of ultrasound as an enhancer for transcutaneous drug delivery: phonophoresis. *Phys Ther*. 1995;75:539–553.
36. Griffin JE, Touchstone JC. Low intensity phonophoresis of cortisol in swine. *Phys Ther*. 1968;48:1336–1344.

ADDITIONAL READINGS

Abramson D, Burnet C, Bell Y, et al. Changes in blood flow, oxygen uptake and tissue temperatures produced by therapeutic physical agents I. Effects of ultrasound. *Am J Phys Med.* 1960;39:51–62.

Aldes JH, Jadeson WJ, Grabinski S. A new approach to the treatment of subdeltoid bursitis. *Am J Phys Med.* 1954;33:79–88.

Aldes JH, Klaras T. Use of ultrasonic radiation in the treatment of subdeltoid bursitis with and without calcareous deposits. *West J Surg, Ob Gyn.* 1954;62:369–376.

Balmaseda MT, Fatehi MT, Koozekanani SH, Lee AL. Ultrasound therapy: a comparative study of different coupling media. *Arch Phys Med Rehabil.* 1986;67:147–150.

Bearzy HJ. Clinical applications of ultrasonic energy in treatment of acute and chronic subacromial bursitis. *Arch Phys Med Rehabil.* 1953;34:228–231.

Binder A, Hodge G, Hazleman BL, Page Thomas DP. Is therapeutic ultrasound effective in treating soft tissue lesions? *Br Med J.* 1985;290:512–514.

Black KD, Halveson JL, Majerus DA, Soderberg GL. Alterations in ankle dorsiflexion torque as a result of continuous ultrasound to the anterior tibial compartment. *Phys Ther.* 1984; 64:910–913.

Bromley J, Unsworth A, Haslock I. Changes in stiffness following short- and long-term application of standard physiotherapeutic techniques. *Br J Rheumatol.* 1994;33:555–561.

Clark GR, Stenner L. Use of therapeutic ultrasound. *Physiotherapy.* 1976;62:185–190.

Coakley WT. Biophysical effect of ultrasound at therapeutic intensities. *Physiotherapy.* 1978;64:166–169.

Cosentino AB, Cross DL, Harrington RJ, Soderberg GL. Ultrasound effects on electroneuromyographic measures in sensory fibers of the median nerve. *Phys Ther.* 1983;63: 1788–1792.

Creates V. A study of ultrasound treatment to the painful perineum after childbirth. *Physiotherapy.* 1987;73:162–165.

DePreux T. Ultrasonic wave therapy in osteoarthritis of the hip joint. *Br J Phys Med.* 1952;15:14–19.

Docker MF. A review of instrumentation available for therapeutic ultrasound. *Physiotherapy.* 1987;73:154–155.

Downing DS, Weinstein A. Ultrasound therapy of subacromial bursitis: a double blind trial. *Phys Ther.* 1986;66:194–199.

Draper DO, Schulthies S, Sorvisto P, Hautala AM. Temperature changes in deep muscles of humans during ice and ultrasound therapies: an *in vivo* study. *J Orthop Sports Phys Ther.* 1995;21:153–157.

Echternach JL. Ultrasound: an adjunct treatment for shoulder disabilities. *Phys Ther.* 1965;45:865–869.

Enwemeka CS. The effects of therapeutic ultrasound on tendon healing: a biomechanical study. *Am J Phys Med Rehabil.* 1989;68:283–287.

Ernst E. Use a new treatment while it still works: ultrasound for epicondylitis. *Eur J Phys Med Rehabil.* 1994;4:50–51.

Fabrizio PA, Schmidt JA, Clemente FR, et al. Acute effects of therapeutic ultrasound delivered at varying parameters on the blood flow velocity in a muscular distribution artery. *J Orthop Sports Phys Ther.* 1996;24:294–302.

Falconer J, Hayes KW, Chang RW. Effect of ultrasound on mobility in osteoarthritis of the knee: a randomized clinical trial. *Arthritis Care Res.* 1992;5:29–35.

Farmer WC. Effect of intensity of ultrasound on conduction of motor axons. *Phys Ther.* 1968;48:1233–1237.

Ferguson B. *A Practitioner's Guide to the Ultrasonic Therapy Equipment Standard.* Rockville, Md: US Department of Health and Human Services. 1985. HHS Publication FDA 85-8240.

Flax HJ. Ultrasound treatment of peritendinitis calcarea of the shoulder. *Am J Phys Med.* 1964;43:117–124.

Frieder S, Weisberg J, Fleming B, Stanek A. A pilot study: the therapeutic effect of ultrasound following partial rupture of Achilles tendons in male rats. *J Orthop Sports Phys Ther.* 1988;10:39–45.

Frizzell LA, Dunn F. Biophysics of ultrasound. In: Lehmann JF, ed. *Therapeutic Heat and Cold.* 3rd ed. Baltimore: Williams & Wilkins; 1982:353–385.

Gam AN, Johannsen F. Ultrasound therapy in musculoskeletal disorders: a meta-analysis. *Pain.* 1995;63:85–91.

Gnatz SM. Increased radicular pain due to therapeutic ultrasound applied to the back. *Arch Phys Med Rehabil.* 1989;70:493–494.

Goddard DH, Revell PA, Cason J, et al. Ultrasound has no anti-inflammatory effect. *Ann Rheum Dis.* 1983;42:582–584.

Gorkiewicz R. Ultrasound for subacromial bursitis: a case report. *Phys Ther.* 1984;64:46–47.

Griffin JE. Transmissiveness of ultrasound through tap water, glycerin, and mineral oil. *Phys Ther.* 1980;60:1010–1016.

Griffin JE, Echternach JL, Bowmaker KL. Results of frequency differences in ultrasonic therapy. *Phys Ther.* 1970;50:481–486.

Grynbaum BB. An evaluation of the clinical use of ultrasonics. *Am J Phys Med.* 1954;33:75–78.

Gulick DT. Effectively using ultrasound. *Rehabil Management.* June/July 1998:46–53.

Hamer J, Kirk JA. Physiotherapy and the frozen shoulder: a comparative trial of ice and ultrasonic therapy. *N Z Med J.* 1976;83:191–192.

Hashish I, Harvey W, Harris M. Anti-inflammatory effects of ultrasound therapy: evidence for a major placebo effect. *Br J Rheumatol.* 1986;25:77–81.

Hayes KW. The use of ultrasound to decrease pain and improve mobility. *Crit Rev Phys Rehabil Med.* 1992;3:271–287.

Hekkenberg RT, Oosterbaan WA, Van Beekum WT. Evaluation of ultrasound therapy devices. *Physiotherapy.* 1986;72:390–395.

Herrick JF. Temperatures produced in tissues by ultrasound: experimental study using various technics. *J Acoust Soc Am.* 1953;25:12–16.

Hill CR, ter Haar G, Suess MJ, ed. Ultrasound. *Nonionizing radiation protection.* Copenhagen: World Health Organization; 1982:199–228.

Imig CJ, Randall BF, Hines HM. Effect of ultrasonic energy on blood flow. *Am J Phys Med.* 1954;33:100–102.

Inaba MK, Piorkowski M. Ultrasound in treatment of painful shoulders in patients with hemiplegia. *Phys Ther.* 1972;52:737–742.

Jan M, Lai J. The effects of physiotherapy on osteoarthritic knees of females. *J Formosan Med Assn.* 1991;90:1008–1013.

Jones RJ. Treatment of acute herpes zoster using ultrasonic therapy: report on a series of twelve patients. *Physiotherapy.* 1984;70:94–96.

Klemp P, Staberg B, Korsgärd J, et al. Reduced blood flow in fibromyotic muscles during ultrasound therapy. *Scand J Rehabil Med.* 1982;15:21–23.

Konrad K. Randomized, double blind, placebo-controlled study of ultrasonic treatment of the hands of rheumatoid arthritis patients. *Eur J Phys Med Rehabil.* 1994;5:155–157.

Kramer JF. Ultrasound: evaluation of its mechanical and thermal effects. *Arch Phys Med Rehabil.* 1984;65:223–227.

Lehmann JF, Brunner GD, Stow RW. Pain threshold measurements after therapeutic application of ultrasound, microwaves and infrared. *Arch Phys Med Rehabil.* 1958;39:560–565.

Lehmann JF, DeLateur BJ, Silvermann DR. Selective heating effects of ultrasound in human beings. *Arch Phys Med Rehabil.* 1966;47:331–339.

Lehmann JF, DeLateur BJ, Warren CG, Stonebridge JB. Heating of joint structures by ultrasound. *Arch Phys Med Rehabil.* 1968;49:28–30.

Lehmann JF, Erickson DJ, Martin GM, Krusen FH. Comparison of ultrasonic and microwave diathermy in the physical treatment of periarthritis of the shoulder. *Arch Phys Med Rehabil.* 1954;35:627–634.

Lehmann JF, Fordyce WE, Rathbun LA, et al. Clinical evaluation of a new approach in the treatment of contracture associated with hip fracture after internal fixation. *Arch Phys Med Rehabil.* 1961;42:95–100.

Lehmann JF, McMillan JA, Brunner GD, Blumberg JB. Comparative study of the efficiency of short-wave, microwave and ultrasonic diathermy in heating the hip joint. *Arch Phys Med Rehabil.* 1959;40:510–512.

Lehmann JF, Stonebridge J, DeLateur BJ, et al. Temperature in human thighs after hot pack treatment followed by ultrasound. *Arch Phys Med Rehabil.* 1978;59:472–475.

Levenson JL, Weissberg MP. Ultrasound abuse: case report. *Arch Phys Med Rehabil.* 1983;64:90–91.

Lowdon A. Application of ultrasound to assess stress fractures. *Physiotherapy.* 1986;72: 160–161.

Lundeberg T, Abrahamsson P, Haker E. A comparative study of continuous ultrasound, placebo ultrasound and rest in epicondylalgia. *Scand J Rehabil Med.* 1988;20:99–101.

MacDonald BL, Shipster SB. Temperature changes induced by continuous ultrasound. *S Afr J Physiother.* 1981;37:13–15.

Madsen PW, Gersten JW. The effect of ultrasound on conduction velocity of peripheral nerve. *Arch Phys Med Rehabil.* 1961;42:645–649.

Magee DJ. Effect of therapeutic ultrasound on human blood sugar. *Physiother Can.* 1983;35:135–138.

McDiarmid T, Burns PN. Clinical applications of therapeutic ultrasound. *Physiotherapy.* 1987;73:155–162.

McDiarmid T, Burns PN, Lewith GT, Machin D. Ultrasound and the treatment of pressure sores. *Physiotherapy.* 1985;71:66–70.

McMeeken J. Tissue temperature and blood flow: a research based overview of electrophysical modalities. *Aust J Physiother.* 1994;40(4):49–57.

Midlemast S, Chatterjee D. Comparison of ultrasound and thermotherapy for soft tissue injuries. *Physiotherapy.* 1978;64:331–332.

Mueller EE, Mead S, Schulz BF, Vaden MR. A placebo-controlled study of ultrasound treatment for periarthritis. *Am J Phys Med.* 1954;33:31–35.

Munting E. Ultrasonic therapy for painful shoulders. *Physiotherapy.* 1978;64:180–181.

Newman MK, Kill M, Frampton G. Effects of ultrasound alone and combined with hydrocortisone injections by needle or hypospray. *Am J Phys Med.* 1958;37:206–209.

Newman MK, Murphy AJ. Application of ultrasonics in chronic rheumatic diseases. *Mich State Med Soc.* 1952; 51:1213–1215.

Nussbaum EL, Biemann I, Mustard B. Comparison of ultrasound/ultraviolet-C and laser for treatment of pressure ulcers in patients with spinal cord injury. *Phys Ther.* 1994;74: 812–825.

Nwuga VCB. Ultrasound in treatment of back pain resulting from prolapsed intervertebral disc. *Arch Phys Med Rehabil.* 1983;64:88–89.

Partridge CJ. Evaluation of the efficacy of ultrasound. *Physiotherapy.* 1987;73:166–168.

Patrick MK. Application of pulsed ultrasound. *Physiotherapy.* 1978;64:103–104.

Payne C. Ultrasound for post-herpetic neuralgia: a study to investigate the results of treatment. *Physiotherapy.* 1984;70:96–97.

Payton OD, Lamb RL, Kasey ME. Effects of therapeutic ultrasound on bone marrow in dogs. *Phys Ther.* 1975;55:20–27.

Perron M, Malouin F. Acetic acid iontophoresis and ultrasound for the treatment of calcifying tendinitis of the shoulder: a randomized control trial. *Arch Phys Med Rehabil.* 1997;78:379–384.

Portwood MM, Lieberman JS, Taylor RG. Ultrasound treatment of reflex sympathetic dystrophy. *Arch Phys Med Rehabil.* 1987;68:116–118.

Quirion-deGirardi C, Seaborne D, Savard-Goulet F, et al. The analgesic effect of high voltage galvanic stimulation combined with ultrasound in the treatment of low back pain: a one-group pretest/post-test study. *Physiother Can.* 1984;36:327–333.

Reed B, Ashikaga T. The effects of heating with ultrasound on knee joint displacement. *J Orthop Sports Phys Ther.* 1997;26:131–137.

Reid DC, Cummings G. Efficiency of ultrasound coupling agents. *Physiotherapy.* 1977; 63:255–257.

Robinson SE, Buono MJ. Effect of continuous-wave ultrasound on blood flow in skeletal muscle. *Phys Ther.* 1995;75:145–150.

Roche C, West J. A controlled trial investigating the effect of ultrasound on venous ulcers referred from general practitioners. *Physiotherapy.* 1984;70:475–477.

Sandler V. The thermal effects of pulsed ultrasound. *S Afr J Physiother.* 1981;37:10–12.

Santiesteban AJ. The role of physical agents in the treatment of spine pain. *Clin Orthop.* 1983;179:24–30.

Skoubo-Kristensen E, Sommer J. Ultrasound influence on internal fixation with a rigid plate in dogs. *Arch Phys Med Rehabil.* 1982;63:371–373.

Stewart HF, Harris GR, Herman BA, et al. Survey of the use and performance of ultrasonic therapy equipment in Pinellas, County, Florida. *Phys Ther.* 1974;54:707–715.

Stratton S, Heckmann R, Francis RS. Therapeutic ultrasound: its effects on the integrity of a nonpenetrating wound. *J Orthop Sports Phys Ther.* 1984;5:278–281.

Svarcová J, Trnavsky K, Zvárová J. The influence of ultrasound, galvanic currents and shortwave diathermy on pain intensity in patients with osteoarthritis. *Scand J Rheumatol.* 1988;67(suppl):83–85.

Szumski AJ. Mechanism of pain relief of therapeutic application of ultrasound. *Phys Ther.* 1960;40:116–119.

Ter Haar G. Basic physics of therapeutic ultrasound. *Physiotherapy.* 1978;64:100–103.

Ter Haar G. Basic physics of therapeutic ultrasound. *Physiotherapy.* 1987;73:110–113.

Vaughen JL, Bender LF. Effects of ultrasound on growing bone. *Arch Phys Med Rehabil.* 1959;40:158–160.

Vaughn DT. Direct method versus underwater method in the treatment of plantar warts with ultrasound. *Phys Ther.* 1973;53:396–397.

Ward AR, Robertson VJ. Comparison of heating of nonliving soft tissue produced by 45 kHz and 1 MHz frequency ultrasound machines. *J Orthop Sports Phys Ther.* 1996;23:258–266.

Warren CG, Koblanski JN, Sigelman RA. Ultrasound coupling media: their relative transmissivity. *Arch Phys Med Rehabil.* 1976;57:218–222.

Wessling KC, DeVane DA, Hylton CR. Effects of static stretch versus static stretch and ultrasound combined on triceps surae muscle extensibility in healthy women. *Phys Ther.* 1987;67:674–679.

Williams R. Production and transmission of ultrasound. *Physiotherapy.* 1987;73:113–116.

Wright EJ, Hasse KH. Keloids and ultrasound. *Arch Phys Med Rehabil.* 1971;52:280–281.

Zankel HT. Effect of physical agents on motor nerve conduction velocity of the ulnar nerve. *Arch Phys Med Rehabil.* 1966;47:787–791.

Phonophoresis

Antich TJ. Phonophoresis: the principles of the ultrasonic driving force and efficacy in treatment of common orthopaedic diagnoses. *J Orthop Sports Phys Ther.* 1982;4:99–102.

Bare AC, McAnaw MB, Pritchard AE, et al. Phonophoretic delivery of 10% hydrocortisone through the epidermis of humans as determined by serum cortisol concentrations. *Phys Ther.* 1996;76:738–749.

Franklin ME, Smith ST, Chenier TC, Franklin RC. Effect of phonophoresis with dexamethasone on adrenal function. *J Orthop Sports Phys Ther.* 1995;22:103–107.

Halle JS, Franklin RJ, Karalfa BL. Comparison of four treatment approaches for lateral epicondylitis of the elbow. *J Orthop Sports Phys Ther.* 1986;8:62–67.

Panus PC, Hooper T, Padrones A, et al. A case study of exacerbation of lateral epicondylitis by combined use of iontophoresis and phonophoresis. *Physiother Can.* 1996;48:27–31.

Santiesteban AJ. The role of physical agents in the treatment of spine pain. *Clin Orthop.* 1983;179:24–30.

Stratford PW, Levy DR, Gauldie S, et al. The evaluation of phonophoresis and friction massage as treatments for extensor carpi radialis tendinitis: a randomized controlled trial. *Physiother Can.* 1989;41:93–99.

Wing M. Phonophoresis with hydrocortisone in the treatment of temporomandibular joint dysfunction. *Phys Ther.* 1982;62:32–33.

Cryotherapy

There are several methods of delivering cold treatments for therapeutic purposes. A general discussion of cold follows, and then each procedure for delivering cold is presented separately.

PURPOSE AND EFFECTS

Cold applications are generally used to diminish physiologic functions such as blood flow, inflammatory response, or muscle activity.

Local Applications

1. Local vasoconstriction with a reduction in blood flow occurs in direct response to cold application.[1,2] Cold-induced vasodilation has been observed in the skin following exposure to extreme cold.[3,4] When a part becomes so cold that the viability of the tissues is threatened, vasodilation results. Some very superficial vasodilation may also occur in response to irritation of sensory nerve endings by extremely cold sources. At the present time, whether this cold-induced vasodilation is therapeutic, inconsequential, or deleterious is yet to be determined. Several investigators have measured temperature in deeper tissues, especially muscle, and have not found any indication of vasodilation during cold treatment.[1,5,6]

2. Local metabolism is decreased, and thus the demand for oxygen is lessened and responses to acute injury or inflammation are decreased.[7]

3. Long-term treatment with cold (>30 minutes) can lower intra-articular temperature, reducing joint metabolism and activity of cartilage-degrading enzymes.[8]

4. Nerve conduction velocity is slowed with eventual conduction failure.[9]

5. Pain threshold is increased.[10,11]
6. Endorphins may be released.[12]
7. Muscle spindle activity is diminished.[13]
8. The ability to perform rapid movements is diminished, perhaps from increased muscle viscosity or from prolonged contraction and relaxation times.[14]
9. Connective tissue becomes stiffer and is not as plastic following a cold treatment. Tensile strength decreases.[15,16]
10. Force generation, both concentric and eccentric, is diminished following ice application.[17,18] Concentric force generation recovers faster than eccentric force generation, especially if moderate exercise is used.[17]

General Applications

1. There is generalized vasoconstriction in response to cooling of the posterior hypothalamus.[19]
2. Respiratory and heart rates are slowed.[20]
3. Muscle tone is increased and may be accompanied by shivering. The increase in muscle spindle bias tends to increase spasticity and is directly opposite of the effect of a local application.[19]
4. If application is prolonged, metabolism is increased to produce heat and maintain homeostasis.[19]

INDICATIONS

1. Spasticity accompanying central nervous system disorders if the increased tone interferes with function.[21] (Be sure treatment is local; the rest of the body should be kept warm.[22,23])
2. Early acute injury or inflammation (e.g., contusions, strains, sprains, postsurgery).[24]
3. Acute or chronic pain (e.g., rheumatoid arthritis, trigger points, acute injury).[25–30]
4. Emergency care for small burns.[31] Cold immersion must be initiated immediately to be effective.[32,33] If the patient is burned extensively, do not use ice; it could result in hypothermia[34] or increased tissue necrosis.[35]
5. Limitation of motion secondary to pain.[27,28,30]
6. Edema (cool sources, in conjunction with elevation).[36]

CONTRAINDICATIONS

1. Patients with angina pectoris or other cardiac dysfunction should not be treated with general cold.[38] Relatively minor problems distant from the thorax may be treated with local cold applications safely.
2. Because of the vasoconstriction produced by cold, open wounds should not be treated after 48 to 72 hours.[39]
3. Patients with arterial insufficiency are at risk for tissue damage from further vasoconstriction with cold exposures.[24]
4. Patients demonstrating hypersensitivity to cold (cold urticaria [hives], Raynaud's phenomenon, fainting) should not be treated.[24,40]

CLINICAL TIP 6–1

Cryokinetics

In the management of most musculoskeletal problems, cold is used to relieve pain or decrease muscle tone to enable the patient to perform other activities. Cryokinetics is the use of a combination of cold treatments and stretching. For acute or subacute injury move the involved part into its pain free end range during the cold treatment while the part is numb. When the numbness is lost, repeat the process, progressing the stretching within the patient's tolerance.[37]

5. Patients with preexisting anesthetic skin cannot report when they become anesthetic from cold. Tissue damage occurs at temperatures only slightly below that which produces anesthesia.
6. Regenerating peripheral nerves are at risk with cold exposures because the tensile strength of the recovering axons is already low.

PRECAUTION

Old people vasoconstrict less efficiently[41] and often do not shiver.[42] Because of this decreased ability to conserve or produce heat, they are not very tolerant of generalized exposures to cold.

DOSAGE

Intensity

The intensity of a cold treatment is directly related to the goal to be achieved. Cold interventions used to reduce swelling and slow metabolism must be mild, or swelling and metabolism may increase.[43] To block pain, the cold source may be very cold.

Duration

The duration of cold treatments depends on the depth of the target tissue, the goal of the treatment, and the temperature of the source. Deeper tissues must be cooled for longer periods than superficial ones. Very cold sources must be used for shorter periods than sources that are merely cool. Specific durations of treatment will be discussed below for each cooling source.

Frequency

Cold procedures may be repeated during each treatment session if they prove helpful. The use of cold for acute injury or in recent wounds, however, should be discontinued after the initial 2 or 3 days, because cold can delay healing.

Ice Packs

DESCRIPTION

An ice pack can be made of crushed ice in the clinic without much expense. It may be used in any condition in which cold is indicated and is a good method to use if prolonged cooling and a very cold source are desired.

INSTRUCTIONS

1. Instruct the patient about what you are going to do, what to expect from the treatment, and what you expect of him. Be sure to describe the sensation cycle (see Responses to Treatment, below).
2. Position the patient for comfort and make sure he is warm.

3. Check the patient's temperature sensation and skin integrity.
4. Prepare the pack as follows:
   a. Fill a plastic bag with crushed ice or small ice cubes. Add a bit of water to lower the temperature further. Bleed the air out of the bag and seal it.
   b. Spread out a large, *moist* terry cloth towel and place the plastic bag in the center.
   c. Fold the edges over to make a pack.
5. Place the pack on the patient, covering the involved muscles or joints and molding the bag to fit the contour of the part. Cover the pack with dry toweling and waterproof covering if necessary to protect the patient's clothing or furniture.
6. The pack may be left in place for 10 to 20 minutes. The time depends on the bulk of the tissues and the depth of the tissue to be cooled. A pack must remain in place longer than 10 minutes if prolonged, deep tissue cooling are desired. Additional packs may be necessary for lengthy treatments.
7. Remove the pack, dry the patient, and check the patient's skin and physiologic responses to the cold treatment.
8. Follow with exercises, if indicated.
9. Perform all appropriate posttreatment evaluation procedures.
10. Document the treatment, including the method used, temperature, area treated, patient position, duration of treatment, and the patient response during and following treatment.

Commercial Cold Packs

DESCRIPTION

Commercial cold packs are generally made of plastic and filled with a hydrated gel. They come in a variety of shapes and sizes and are reusable. These packs are kept in a refrigeration unit or home freezer at 0°F to 10°F (−21°C to −12°C). They are pliable and neat, and although they maintain their low temperature for an extended period, they do not lower skin temperature as much as ice does. They can be used for any condition in which cold is indicated, especially if less intense, prolonged cooling is desired. Achievement of actual anesthesia with these packs is doubtful.

INSTRUCTIONS

1. Before beginning treatment, be sure to check the temperature of the freezer unit to be sure that the packs are at the anticipated temperature.
2. Instruct the patient about the treatment, what to expect, and what you expect of her. Check for temperature sensation and skin integrity.
3. Position and drape the patient appropriately. Be sure to keep the rest of the body warm, because only local effects are desired.
4. Cover the involved area with a single layer of moist toweling. Moisture

is necessary to enhance the heat exchange between the pack and the patient. To diminish the initial shock of the cold treatment, the towel may be warm when applied.

5. Place the pack over the towel, molding it to fit the part. Cover the pack with several layers of dry toweling.
6. Treatment time is 10 to 20 minutes for treatments aimed at controlling edema, pain, or bleeding. Treatments up to several hours are acceptable in emergency situations such as immediately following a burn. The use of additional packs may become necessary for prolonged treatment to maintain the thermal gradient between the pack and the patient.
7. Remove the pack, dry the patient, and check skin condition and general physiologic responses.
8. Follow with exercises, if indicated.
9. Perform other posttreatment evaluations appropriate for the patient.
10. Document the treatment, including the method used, temperature, area treated, patient position, duration of treatment, and patient response during and following treatment.

Ice Massage

DESCRIPTION

This procedure involves rubbing a large cube of ice over the involved area of the patient's body. An easy way to obtain these cubes is by freezing water in paper or plastic foam cups or juice cans in which lollipop sticks have been placed. The cubes should be round, because sharp edges can be irritating. Regardless of how the cubes are made, ice massage is most appropriate for small areas of painful muscle guarding and for acute injuries to decrease pain, edema, and hemorrhage. This procedure decreases temperature rapidly, and with sufficient time, it can decrease intramuscular temperature.[44]

INSTRUCTIONS

1. Instruct the patient regarding what you are going to do, what to expect from the treatment, and what you expect of him. Be sure to describe the sensation cycle (see Responses to Treatment, below).
2. Position the patient appropriately. All unnecessary clothing should be removed, because the treatment is messy. Drape carefully and have extra towels available. It is important to keep the patient warm, because only local effects are desired.
3. Check the patient's temperature sensation and skin integrity.
4. Provide verbal support throughout the treatment, and be sure to warn the patient at the onset of treatment.
5. Remove the ice lollipop from its container and begin rubbing the ice over the painful area. Use a moderate speed and rhythmic motion. For very small areas, the tip of the lollipop works best, whereas the sides of the lollipop work better for larger areas. Be sure to blot up any water as it forms.

6. Continue the application until anesthesia is reached. This usually occurs within 5 to 10 minutes.
7. Dry the patient, and check his skin condition and general physiologic responses.
8. Follow with exercises, if indicated.
9. Perform other posttreatment evaluation procedures appropriate for the patient.
10. Document the treatment, including method used, temperature, area treated, patient position, duration of treatment, and patient response during and following treatment.

Cold Baths (Immersion)

DESCRIPTION

Immersion involves placing the part to be treated in water ranging in temperature from cool to icy. The temperature ranges most commonly used are summarized in Table 6–1. This method is appropriate for treatment of an extremity or for large body areas; the temperature of the water depends on the condition. When considering selection of this technique, remember that the part treated must be in a dependent position. Thus, this may not be the treatment of choice if the condition involves distal swelling.

INSTRUCTIONS

1. Instruct the patient about what you are going to do, what to expect from treatment, and what you expect of her. Check temperature sensation and skin integrity.
2. Fill a pail or whirlpool to an appropriate level with water of the desired temperature. To make treatments with cold and very cold temperatures more comfortable for the patient, lower the temperature gradually by adding cold water or ice until the desired temperature is reached. The greater the body area immersed, the warmer the water must be.
3. Position the patient so that she may comfortably put the extremity into the water. If cool baths are being used to decrease spasticity in prepara-

TABLE 6–1. Temperature Ranges Commonly Used With Ice Immersions		
DESCRIPTOR	°F	°C*
Cool	67.0–80.0	19.0–27.0
Cold	55.0–67.0	13.0–19.0
Very Cold	32.0–55.0	0.0–13.0

* Degrees Celcius are rounded to the nearest half degree.

tion for gait activities, a standing position might be considered. Be sure to keep the rest of the patient's body warm.

4. If the bath is used for pain relief, the part treated should remain immersed in very cold water until anesthesia is reached. Treatments in cool water for spasticity or inflammation may last for 10 to 20 minutes.
5. Dry the patient and check her skin and physiologic response to the cold treatment.
6. Follow with exercises, if indicated.
7. Perform all other appropriate posttreatment evaluation procedures.
8. Document the treatment, including method used, temperature, area treated, patient position, duration of treatment, and the patient response during and following treatment.

Vapocoolant Spray

DESCRIPTION

Vapocoolants such as ethyl chloride or fluoromethane sprays are highly volatile liquids that produce significant cooling through evaporation when sprayed on the skin. The spray is contained in a glass bottle equipped with a nozzle capable of ejecting a fine stream. Vapocoolants are particularly effective in reducing painful muscle guarding and desensitizing trigger areas. Ethyl chloride is often used today by physicians to anesthetize a skin surface prior to injection with steroid medication.

Concern has been raised that chlorofluorocarbons damage the ozone layer, allowing biologically hazardous wavelengths of ultraviolet radiation to reach the earth.[45] Even though medical use of vapocoolants contributes little to the atmospheric damage and the risk of skin cancer from ultraviolet radiation, the efficacy of the vapocoolants in comparison with other cooling agents has not been established. Although vapocoolants have been used frequently with trigger points, other methods of cooling such as ice massage are available to practitioners.

Ethyl chloride, particularly, is hazardous for other reasons. It produces greater levels of cooling, can be dangerous to the skin, is flammable and explosive, and can act as a general anesthetic if the vapors accumulate.[46] Because of the danger to the atmosphere and the inherent hazards associated with the use of vapocoolants, they should be avoided when possible.

INSTRUCTIONS

1. Instruct the patient regarding what to expect from treatment and what you expect of him. Check for temperature sensation and skin condition.
2. Position the patient for comfort and accessibility of the part to be treated. Be sure the rest of the patient's body is warm. If treatment is to be near the face, provide some means of shielding it to protect the patient's eyes from the spray as well as to prevent inhalation of the vapor.

3. Remove all sources of ignition from the treatment area, because some of the vapocoolant sprays are highly flammable.[47]
4. Hold the container, nozzle down, about 2 ft (52 cm) from the patient in such a way that the stream strikes the surface on an angle.[47,48]
5. Spray the painful area in one direction only, moving at a rate of about 4 in. (1.6 cm)/sec.[48] Allow the spray to evaporate completely before starting the next sweep. Be careful not to frost the skin.[47]
6. Cover the entire area one or two times with adjacent rhythmic sweeps. When treating trigger areas, treat both the trigger area and the reference zone.[47]
7. For patients who have limitation of motion, while you are spraying, take the part through passive range of motion, stretching slightly at the end of range.[47] Have the patient perform active motion immediately after spraying.
8. The entire series of sprays may be repeated, if desired, for a good result.
9. Stop treatment if no effect is evident within 5 minutes.[47]
10. Perform all appropriate posttreatment evaluation procedures, including skin inspection.
11. Document the treatment, including method used, temperature, area treated, patient position, duration of treatment, and patient response during and following treatment.

Contrast Baths

DESCRIPTION

Contrast baths are immersions of body parts in baths in which both warm and cold water temperatures are used alternately.

PURPOSE AND EFFECTS

Contrast applications are primarily used as a type of "vascular exercise," causing alternate constriction and dilation of the local blood vessels. The alternation stimulates peripheral blood flow and helps stimulate healing. Both the heat and the cold produce effects that have been discussed in their respective sections, but the adverse effects of each are less likely to occur. For example, edema, which would be aggravated by the use of heat, is discouraged by the presence of the cold.

INDICATIONS

Contrast baths have been used for the following conditions, but few studies have been performed to support the efficacy of use for these problems.[24,49,50]

1. Impaired venous circulation.
2. Subacute or chronic traumatic and inflammatory conditions (can be used during the transition period between acute and subacute phases).

3. Edema.
4. Sinus or congestive headaches—applied to the feet or to both the feet and hands to increase peripheral circulation and shunt the blood from the head.

CONTRAINDICATIONS

Because contrast baths use both heat and cold, the risks of both heat and cold apply. Please refer to the contraindications for hydrotherapy and those for cold applications.

PRECAUTIONS

1. Patients with anesthetic skin are not good judges of temperature sensations.
2. Patients who are very young or very old may have inefficient thermoregulatory systems.

INSTRUCTIONS

1. Instruct the patient about what to expect from treatment and what you expect of her.
2. Check for temperature sensation and skin integrity.
3. Position the patient comfortably and appropriately.
4. Drape if necessary and provide linen as needed. Be sure to keep the rest of the patient's body warm.
5. Prepare two pails of water to a depth that covers the area to be treated.
   a. Warm bath: 100°F to 110°F (38°C to 43°C).
   b. Cold bath: 55°F to 65°F (13°C to 18°C).
6. The temperature is selected based on the patient's condition. Extremes of temperature, over 105°F (41°C) or under 65°F (18°C), should be avoided if peripheral circulatory problems are involved. If open wounds are present, a disinfectant such as povidone-iodine or sodium hypochlorite should be added to the water.
7. Immerse the part or parts in the warm bath for 6 minutes.[51]
8. Immerse the part in the cold bath for 4 minutes.[51] If the patient does not tolerate a 4-minute cold immersion, immerse the part long enough to produce vasoconstriction,[50] for at least 1 minute.
9. Repeat steps 6 and 7 so that the total treatment time is 20 to 30 minutes.
10. The treatment may end in either hot or cold, depending on the condition treated (e.g., for edema, ending in cold may be more beneficial).
11. Dry the patient and allow her to rest, or follow with exercises as indicated.
12. Perform all appropriate posttreatment evaluations, including measurement of vital signs and skin inspection.
13. Document the treatment, including method used, temperature, duration of both heat and cold phases, area treated, patient position, and patient response during and following treatment.

RESPONSES TO TREATMENT AND TREATMENT MODIFICATION

The sensations experienced by the patient are predictable and usually appear in 7 to 15 minutes in the following sequence: cold, burning, aching, numbness.[25,26,52] *The complete sequence will occur only with extremely cold sources.* In monitoring skin response, look for excessive redness, swelling, or areas of pallor. These responses may indicate areas of cold injury. If they appear, rewarm the area rapidly, document the occurrence, and file an incident report as appropriate for the facility.

HOME USE

Many cold treatments may be given at home. Ice packs, ice massage, ice baths, contrast baths, and commercial packs are all easily used by the patient at home. Patients should not use vapocoolant sprays at home because of their hazards. Be sure to instruct the patient about construction of the cold source, the temperature at which it should be used, the area to be treated, the dosage for treatment, the responses to anticipate, what to do in the event of a negative response, and how to store the cold source between treatments.

REFERENCES

1. Taber C, Contryman K, Fahrenbruch J, et al. Measurement of reactive vasodilation during cold gel pack application to nontraumatized ankles. *Phys Ther.* 1992;72: 294–299.
2. Thorsson O, Lilja B, Ahlgren L, et al. The effect of local cold application on intramuscular blood flow at rest and after running. *Med Sci Sports Exerc.* 1985;17:710–713.
3. Lewis T. Observations upon the reactions of the vessels of the human skin to cold. *Heart.* 1930;15:177–208.
4. Daanan HA, Van de Linde FJ, Romet TT, Ducharme MB. The effect of body temperature on the hunting response of the middle finger skin temperature. *Eur J Appl Physiol.* 1997;76:538–543.
5. Knight KL, Aquino J, Johannes SM, Urban C. A reexamination of Lewis' cold-induced vasodilatation in the fingers and the ankle. *Athletic Training.* 1980;15:248–250.
6. Walton M, Roestenburg M, Hallwright S, Sutherland JC. Effects of ice packs on tissue temperatures at various depths before and after quadriceps hematoma: studies using sheep. *J Orthop Sports Phys Ther.* 1986;8:294–300.
7. Schoessler M, Ludwig-Beymer P, Heuther SE. Pain, temperature regulation, sleep and sensory function. In: McCance KL, Heuther SE, eds. *Pathophysiology: The Biologic Basis for Disease in Adults and Children.* St. Louis: Mosby; 1990:390–430.
8. Kern H, Fessl L, Trnavsky G, Hertz H. Cryotherapy. Behavior of joint temperature during ice application—a basis for practical use. *Wien Klin Wochenschr.* 1984;96:832–837.
9. Lee JM, Warren MP, Mason SM. Effects of ice on nerve conduction velocity. *Physiotherapy.* 1978;64:2–6.
10. Benson TB, Copp EP. The effects of therapeutic forms of heat and ice on the pain threshold of the normal shoulder. *Rheumatol Rehabil.* 1974;13:101–104.
11. Curkovic B, Vitulic V, Babic-Naglic D, Dürrigl T. The influence of heat and cold on the pain threshold in rheumatoid arthritis. *Z Rheumatol.* 1993;52:289–291.
12. Utsinger PD, Bonner F, Hogan N. Efficacy of cryotherapy (CR) and thermotherapy in the management of rheumatoid arthritis (RA) pain: evidence for an endorphin effect. *Arthritis Rheumatol.* 1982;25:S113.

13. Knutsson E. On effects of local cooling upon motor functions in spastic paresis. *Prog Phys Ther.* 1970;1:124–131.

14. Lightfoot E, Verrier M, Ashby P. Neurological effects of prolonged cooling of the calf in patients with complete spinal transection. *Phys Ther.* 1975;55:251–258.

15. Bäcklund L, Tiselius P. Objective measurement of joint stiffness in rheumatoid arthritis. *Acta Rheum Scand.* 1967;13:275–288.

16. Wright V, Johns RJ. Quantitative and qualitative analysis of joint stiffness in normal subjects and in patients with connective tissue diseases. *Ann Rheum Dis.* 1961;20:36–46.

17. Ruiz DH, Myrer JW, Durrant E, Fellingham GW. Cryotherapy and sequential exercise bouts following cryotherapy on concentric and eccentric strength in the quadriceps. *J Athletic Training.* 1993;28:320–323.

18. Cornwall MW. Effect of temperature on muscle force and rate of muscle force production in men and women. *J Orthop Sports Phys Ther.* 1994;20:74–80.

19. Guyton AC. *Human Physiology and Mechanisms of Disease.* 5th ed. Philadelphia: W.B. Saunders; 1992.

20. LeBlanc J, Blais B, Barabe B, Côté J. Effects of temperature and wind on facial temperature, heart rate, and sensation. *J Appl Physiol.* 1976;40:127–131.

21. Chan CWY. Some techniques for the relief of spasticity and their physiological basis. *Physiother Can.* 1986;38:85–89.

22. Newton MJ, Lehmkuhl D. Muscle spindle responses to body heating and localized muscle cooling. *Phys Ther.* 1965;45:91–105.

23. DonTigny RL, Sheldon KW. Simultaneous use of heat and cold in treatment of muscle spasm. *Arch Phys Med Rehabil.* 1962;49:308–314.

24. Lehmann JF, DeLateur BJ. Cryotherapy (pp. 563–602). In Lehmann JF, ed. *Therapeutic Heat and Cold.* 3rd ed. Baltimore: Williams & Wilkins; 1982.

25. Grant A. Massage with ice (cryokinetics) in the treatment of painful conditions of the musculoskeletal system. *Arch Phys Med Rehabil.* 1964;45:233–238.

26. Hayden C. Cryokinetics in an early treatment program. *Phys Ther.* 1964;44:990–993.

27. Halliday Pegg SM, Littler TR, Littler MD. A trial of ice therapy and exercise in chronic arthritis. *Physiotherapy.* 1969;55:51–56.

28. Kangilaski J. 'Baggietherapy': simple pain relief for arthritic knees. *JAMA.* 1981;246:317–318.

29. Kirk JA, Kersley GD. Heat and cold in the physical treatment of rheumatoid arthritis of the knee. *Ann Phys Med.* 1968;9:270–274.

30. Chambers R. Clinical uses of cryotherapy. *Phys Ther.* 1969;49:245–249.

31. Settle JAD. Burns: emergency treatment and resuscitation. *Physiotherapy.* 1977;63:146–150.

32. Raine TJ, Heggers JP, Robson MC, et al. Cooling the burn wound to maintain microcirculation. *J Trauma.* 1981;21:394–397.

33. Demling RH, Mazess RB, Wolberg W. The effect of immediate and delayed cold immersion on burn edema formation and resorption. *J Trauma.* 1979;19:56–60.

34. Wagner MM. Emergency care of the burned patient. *Am J Nurs.* November 1977;1788–1791.

35. Helm PA, Kevorkian CG, Lusbaugh M, et al. Burn injury: rehabilitation management in 1982. *Arch Phys Med Rehabil.* 1982;63:6–16.

36. Michlovitz A, Smith W, Watkins M. Ice and high voltage pulsed stimulation in treatment of acute lateral ankle sprains. *J Orthop Sports Phys Ther.* 1988;9:301–304.

37. Pincivero D, Gieck JH, Saliba EN. Rehabilitation of a lateral ankle sprain with cryokinetics and functional progressive exercise. *J Sport Rehabil.* 1993;2:200–207.

38. Stanghelle JK, Nilsson S. Angina pectoris and cold. *Int Rehabil Med.* 1983;5:189–191.

39. Lundgren C, Muren A, Zederfeldt B. Effect of cold-vasoconstriction on wound healing in rabbit. *Acta Chir Scand.* 1959;118:1–4.

40. Delp HL, Newton RA. Effects of brief cold exposure on finger dexterity and sensibility in subjects with Raynaud's phenomenon. *Phys Ther.* 1986;66:503–507.

41. Collins JC, Dore C, Exton-Smith AN, et al. Accidental hypothermia and impaired temperature homeostasis in the elderly. *Br Med J.* 1977;1:353–356.

42. LeBlanc J, Côté J, Dulac S, Dulong-Turcot F. Effects of age, sex, and physical fitness on responses to local cooling. *J Appl Physiol.* 1978;44:813–817.
43. Coté DJ, Prentice WE, Hooker DN, Shields EW. Comparison of three treatment procedures for minimizing ankle sprain swelling. *Phys Ther.* 1988;68:1072–1076.
44. Zemke JE, Andersen JC, Guion WK, et al. Intramuscular temperature responses in the human leg to two forms of cryotherapy: ice massage and ice bag. *J Orthop Sports Phys Ther.* 1998;27:301–307.
45. Vallentyne SW, Vallentyne JR. The case of the missing ozone: are physiatrists to blame? *Arch Phys Med Rehabil.* 1988;69:992–993.
46. Simons DG, Travell JG, Simons LS. Suggestions: alternate spray; alternative treatments. *Am Phys Ther Assoc Prog Rep.* 1989;18(3):2.
47. Travell J, Rinzler SH. The myofascial genesis of pain. *Postgrad Med.* 1952;11:425–434.
48. Travell J. Ethyl chloride for painful muscle spasm. *Arch Phys Med.* 1952;33:291–298.
49. Engel JP, Wakim KG, Erickson DJ, Krusen FH. The effect of contrast baths on the peripheral circulation of patients with rheumatoid arthritis. *Arch Phys Med.* 1950;31:135–144.
50. Moor FB, Peterson SC, Manwell EM, et al. *Manual of Hydrotherapy and Masssage.* Mountain View, Calif: Pacific Press; 1964.
51. Woodmansey A, Collins DH, Ernst MM. Vascular reactions to the contrast bath in health and in rheumatoid arthritis. *Lancet.* 1938;2:1350–1353.
52. Waylonis GW. The physiologic effects of ice massage. *Arch Phys Med Rehabil.* 1967;48:37–42.

ADDITIONAL READINGS

Amundson H. Thermotherapy and cryotherapy: effects on joint degeneration in rheumatoid arthritis. *Physiother Can.* 1979;31:258–262.
Arledge R. Treatment of patients with frostbite. *Phys Ther.* 1973;53:267–268.
Basset S, Lake B. Use of cold applications in the management of spasticity. *Phys Ther Rev.* 1958;38:333–334.
Borken N, Bierman W. Temperature changes produced by spraying with ethyl chloride. *Arch Phys Med Rehabil.* 1955;36:288–290.
Boynton B, Garramone P, Buca J. Observations of the effects of cool baths for patients with multiple sclerosis. *Phys Ther Rev.* 1959;39:297–299.
Bugaj R. The cooling, analgesic and rewarming effects of ice massage on localized skin. *Phys Ther.* 1975;55:11–19.
Clarke GR, Willis LA, Stenner L, Nichols PJR. Evaluation of physiotherapy in the treatment of osteoarthrosis of the knee. *Rheumatol Rehabil.* 1974;13:190–197.
Conaway B. Ice packs in diabetic neuropathy. *Phys Ther Rev.* 1961;41:586–588.
Dervin GF, Taylor DE, Keene GCR. Effects of cold and compression dressings on early postoperative outcomes for the arthroscopic anterior cruciate ligament reconstruction patient. *J Orthop Sports Phys Ther.* 1998;27:403–406.
Dorwart BB, Hansell JR, Schumacher HR. Effects of cold and heat on urate crystal-induced synovitis in the dog. *Arthritis Rheum.* 1974;17:563–571.
Downey JA, Darling RC, Miller JM. The effects of heat, cold, and exercise on the peripheral circulation. *Arch Phys Med Rehabil.* 1968;49:308–314.
Draper DO, Schulthies S, Sorvisto P, Hautala AM. Temperature changes in deep muscles of humans during ice and ultrasound therapies: an *in vivo* study. *J Orthop Sports Phys Ther.* 1995;21:153–157.
Halkovich LR, Personius WJ, Clamann HP, Newton RA. Effect of Fluori-methane spray on passive hip flexion. *Phys Ther.* 1981;61:185–189.
Hamer J, Kirk JA. Physiotherapy and the frozen shoulder: a comparative trial of ice and ultrasonic therapy. *N Z Med J.* 1976;83:191–192.
Hecht PJ, Bachmann S, Booth RE, Rothman RH. Effects of thermal therapy on rehabilitation after total knee arthroplasty. *Clin Orthop.* 1983;178:198–201.
Helliwell P, Wallace F, Evard F. Smoking and ice therapy in rheumatoid arthritis. *Physiotherapy.* 1989;75:551–552.

Hollander JL, Horvath SM. The influence of physical therapy procedures on the intra-articular temperature of normal and arthritic subjects. *Am J Med Sci.* 1949;218:543–548.

Hurley MV, Jones DW, Newham DJ. Arthrogenic quadriceps inhibition and rehabilitation of patients with extensive traumatic knee injuries. *Clin Sci.* 1994;86:305–310.

Jahanshahi M, Pitt P, Williams I. Pain avoidance in rheumatoid arthritis. *J Psychosom Res.* 1989;33:579–589.

Johnson DJ, Moore S, Moore J, Oliver RA. Effects of cold submersion on intramuscular temperature of the gastrocnemius muscle. *Phys Ther.* 1979;59:1238–1242.

Kelly M. Effectiveness of a cryotherapy technique on spasticity. *Phys Ther.* 1969;49:349–353.

Kowal MA. Review of physiological effects of cryotherapy. *J Orthop Sports Phys Ther.* 1983;5:66–73.

Lentell G, Hetherington T, Eagan J, Morgan M. The use of thermal agents to influence the effectiveness of a low-load prolonged stretch. *J Orthop Sports Phys Ther.* 1992;6:200–207.

Leroux A, Bélanger M, Boucher JP. Pain effect on monosynaptic and polysynaptic reflex inhibition. *Arch Phys Med Rehabil.* 1995;76:576–582.

Lewis M, Clayfield J. Temperature changes following quick icing: a brief investigation. *Aust J Physiother.* 1981;27:175–178.

Lowdon B, Moore R. Determinants and nature of intramuscular temperature changes during cold therapy. *Am J Phys Med.* 1975;54:223–233.

Marshall HC, Gregory RT. Cold hypersensitivity: a simple method for its reduction. *Arch Phys Med Rehabil.* 1974;55:119–124.

McMaster WC. A literary review on ice therapy in injuries. *Am J Sports Med.* 1977;5:124–126.

McMeeken J, Lewis MM, Cocks S. Effects of cooling with simulated ice on skin temperature and nerve conduction velocity. *Aust J Physiother.* 1984;30:111–114.

Mennell JM. The therapeutic use of cold. *J Am Osteopath Assoc.* 1975;74:1146/81–1158/93.

Miller CR, Webers RL. The effects of ice massage on an individual's pain tolerance level to electrical stimulation. *J Orthop Sports Phys Ther.* 1990;12:105–109.

Minor MA, Sanford MK. Physical interventions in the management of pain in arthritis: an overview for research and practice. *Arthritis Care Res.* 1993;6:197–206.

Murphy K. The combination of ice and intermittent compression system in the treatment of soft tissue injuries. *Physiotherapy.* 1988;74:41.

Newton RA. Effects of vapocoolants on passive hip flexion in healthy subjects. *Phys Ther.* 1985;65:1034–1036.

Nicholas JJ. Physical modalities in rheumatological rehabilitation. *Arch Phys Med Rehabil.* 1994;75:994–1001.

Nielson AJ. Spray and stretch for pain. *Phys Ther.* 1978;58:567–568.

Olson JE, Stravino VD. A review of cryotherapy. *Phys Ther.* 1972;52:840–853.

Oosterveld FGJ, Rasker JJ. Effects of local heat and cold treatment on surface and articular temperature of arthritic knees. *Arthritis Rheum.* 1994;37:1578–1582.

Oosterveld FGJ, Rasker JJ. Treating arthritis with locally applied heat or cold. *Semin Arthritis Rheum.* 1994;24:82–90.

Oosterveld FGJ, Rasker JJ, Jacobs JWG, Overmars HJA. The effect of local heat and cold therapy on the intraarticular and skin surface temperature of the knee. *Arthritis Rheum.* 1992;35:146–151.

Prentice WE. An electromyographic analysis of the effectiveness of heat or cold and stretching for inducing relaxation in injured muscle. *J Orthop Sports Phys Ther.* 1982;3:133–140.

Quillen WS, Rouillier LH. Initial management of acute ankle sprains with rapid pulsed pneumatic compression and cold. *J Orthop Sports Phys Ther.* 1982;4:39–43.

Rembe EC. Use of cryotherapy on the post-surgical rheumatoid hand. *Phys Ther.* 1970;50:19–23.

Rockefeller L. The use of cold packs for increasing joint range of motion: a study. *Phys Ther Rev.* 1958;38:564–566.

Salmon J. Physiotherapy in intramuscular lesions. *Aust J Physiother.* 1972;18:18–22.

Stangel L. The value of cryotherapy and thermotherapy in the relief of pain. *Physiother Can.* 1975;27:135–139.

Urbscheit N, Johnston R. Effects of cooling on the ankle jerk and h-response in hemiplegic patients. *Phys Ther.* 1971;51:983–990.

Walters CE, Garrison L, Duncan HJ, et al. The effects of therapeutic agents on muscular strength and endurance. *Phys Ther Rev.* 1960;40:266–270.

Williams J, Harvey J, Tannenbaum H. Use of superficial heat versus ice for the rheumatoid arthritic shoulder: a pilot study. *Physiother Can.* 1986;38:8–13.

Wise DD. Ice and the athlete. *Physiother Can.* 1973;25:213–217.

Wolf BA. Effects of temperature reduction on multiple sclerosis. *Phys Ther.* 1970;50: 808–812.

Wolf SL, Basmajian JV. Intramuscular temperature changes deep to localized cutaneous cold stimulation. *Phys Ther.* 1973;53:1284–1288.

chapter 7

Ultraviolet Radiation

DESCRIPTION

Ultraviolet is radiant energy in the wavelength band of 180 to 400 nm (see Appendix A). This band is further subdivided into four bands as listed in Table 7–1. All the ultraviolet wavelengths are produced by the sun. Those shorter than 290 nm are absorbed by the atmosphere and are available for therapeutic use from artificial sources only. Wavelengths in the UVB and UVC bands penetrate only the epidermis, and UVA wavelengths penetrate to the dermis. In general, ultraviolet waves produce photochemical reactions where they are absorbed. However, the effects may be apparent in tissues other than the absorbing tissue. UVA wavelengths may be able to produce photobiological effects via the circulation.[1]

Three common types of generators are available for use. The air-cooled, high-pressure mercury vapor lamp is one of the common ultraviolet generators. It consists of a quartz tube that permits transmission of the waves. Within the tube is an atmosphere of argon gas in which some mercury has been placed. When an electric current is passed through the generator, the mercury is vapor-

TABLE 7–1. Wavelength Bands of Ultraviolet Radiation

BAND	WAVELENGTHS (NM)
UVA1	340–400
UVA2	320–340
UVB	290–320
UVC	180–290

ized by the resultant heat and emits visible violet and ultraviolet wavelengths in all four ultraviolet bands. The generator is mounted in a reflector that serves to direct the rays to the part to be treated. Shutters are provided to protect the eyes while the burner is lit, because ultraviolet can cause keratitis and conjunctivitis in the unprotected eye. This generator operates at high temperatures and is cooled by circulating air, so it has come to be called a "hot quartz" generator.

The other type of generator available is called a "cold quartz" generator. This type operates in much the same manner as a "hot quartz" generator but at low temperatures. Its output is confined to the wavelengths of the UVC band. Because of its small size and low heat output, the "cold quartz" generator is portable, handy for bedside care, and may be used at short distances.

A third source of ultraviolet waves is a specially designed fluorescent tube. This tube is a low-pressure lamp that is coated inside with a phosphor that absorbs ultraviolet light and reemits long wavelengths in the UVA region. It can be coupled with filters to increase the specificity of the emitted wavelengths. Usually, multiple tubes are used together in a cabinet to irradiate several body surfaces at once. Most commonly, these tubes are used in the treatment of psoriasis, and the cabinets are found most often in dermatologists' offices. Physical therapists do not use this type of generator, and it is not discussed further.

PURPOSE AND EFFECTS

All effects of ultraviolet waves have a latent period of at least 1 hour. Specific effects are determined by specific wavelengths.

Local Effects

1. Erythema is produced by the release of a vasodilator substance in the epidermis that diffuses to the dermal capillaries and can prove beneficial to wound healing.
2. The production of new cells in the stratum basale is stimulated, thickening the epidermis and hastening healing.
3. Desquamation of epidermal cells is encouraged and is beneficial in the treatment of acne vulgaris.
4. Pigmentation is produced from the conversion of tyrosine to melanin in the stratum basale.
5. Bacteria are destroyed, an effect that is useful in cleansing infected wounds.

General Effects

1. Vitamin D is formed from the skin prohormone 7-dehydrocholesterol in the epidermis.[2]
2. The threshold of the reticuloendothelial cells in the deep epidermis is lowered so that they produce more antibodies in the presence of bacteria, thus tending to increase resistance to infection.[3]

Wavelengths Responsible for the Physiologic Effects

1. Erythema with pigmentation: 290 to 300 nm, with a peak at 297 nm.

2. Erythema without pigmentation: 240 to 260 nm, with a peak at 254 nm.
3. Formation of vitamin D: 270 to 300 nm.
4. Destruction of bacteria: 260 to 270 nm, with a peak at 266 nm and a weaker band at 290 to 310 nm.
5. Reticuloendothelial stimulation: 290 to 400 nm.

In selecting a generator to be used for treatment, the spectra of the generators available must be known. The hot quartz generator produces a wide spectrum throughout the ultraviolet range with peaks of high output at certain wavelengths. In contrast, 90% of the output of the cold quartz generator is of the 254-nm wavelength. This wavelength is somewhat bactericidal and produces a nonpigmenting erythema that may be beneficial in the treatment of wounds. Generators should be selected or purchased based on the compatibility of the output spectrum with the treatment goals.

INDICATIONS

Ultraviolet radiation has been used for many years in the treatment of wounds and skin conditions. Although there is some evidence for its effectiveness in these situations, other methods such as medications and dressings that are more effective or more easily administered have been developed. As a result, ultraviolet radiation is used very little clinically except in dermatology.

Local Treatment

1. To dry the skin and produce exfoliation in acne vulgaris. With the advent of good medications to manage this condition, ultraviolet is now rarely used.
2. To decrease the bacterial load in local pressure sores and other slow-healing wounds, especially if treatment follows pulsed lavage.[4] Pressure ulcers on patients following spinal cord injury respond positively to UVC combined with ultrasound.[5] The efficacy of ultraviolet in wound healing has not been well established; consequently, the treatment is not currently recommended by the Agency for Health Care Policy and Research.[6]

General Treatment

1. Established psoriasis. Broad-spectrum ultraviolet treatments have been useful, but treatment with UVA and a photosensitizing agent, 8-methoxy psoralen (PUVA) has been especially successful.[7] Performance of PUVA treatments uses exposure booths equipped with UVA-emitting fluorescent tubes.
2. Uremic pruritis.[8]

CONTRAINDICATIONS

1. Acute pulmonary tuberculosis may be exacerbated.[3,9]
2. Patients with cardiac, kidney, or liver disease may not tolerate ultraviolet radiation well.[3,10]

3. Patients who are hyperthyroid or have diabetes mellitus may develop severe itching if given general exposures of ultraviolet radiation.[3,11]
4. Acute eczema or dermatitis may be exacerbated with local exposures.[3,9,12]
5. Systemic lupus erythematosus may be exacerbated by UVB wavelengths.[12,13] These patients may actually benefit from exposure to UVA1. This treatment, however, is still experimental.[1,14,15]
6. Patients with a fever should not be treated.[3]
7. Patients receiving x-ray therapy should not receive ultraviolet radiation to the same area for 3 months. The skin is devitalized, and ultraviolet could cause skin carcinoma. The use of ultraviolet could also decrease the effectiveness of the x-ray therapy.[3]

PRECAUTIONS

1. Some patients are photosensitive as a result of certain conditions or drugs and may manifest general dermatitis and itching following exposure to ultraviolet radiation. The effects of both the ultraviolet and the drug may be enhanced. Routinely check the patient's medical record prior to treatment or question the patient for the following photosensitizers, but be aware that their presence does not guarantee that the patient will be photosensitive.
   a. Drugs such as sulfonamides, tetracyclines, and quinolones (for bacterial infections), psoralens (for psoriasis), gold salts (for rheumatoid arthritis), amiodarone HCl and quinidines (for cardiac arrhythmia), and phenothiazines (for anxiety).[16] When in doubt about any drug, consult a *Physician's Desk Reference*[16] or a pharmacologist.
   b. Syphilis.[11]
   c. Alcohol.[12]
   d. Heat applications immediately before ultraviolet exposure.[17]
   e. Some foods such as strawberries, eggs, or shellfish.[3]
   f. Elevated levels of estrogen.[12]
2. Chronic exposure to ultraviolet radiation has been implicated in the development of skin cancers. The wavelengths in the UVA band are associated with melanoma; UVB can convert keratoses (precancerous skin lesions) to nonmelanoma skin cancers (i.e., squamous cell and basal cell carcinoma).[18]

INSTRUCTIONS

Ultraviolet may be given in general, tonic doses or in small, local doses. Each type is discussed separately; however, some general statements should be made pertaining to the use of ultraviolet, regardless of the procedure.

General Procedures

1. The treatment room should be well ventilated in addition to being warm and private. Ozone, a mildly poisonous gas, is produced in the early warm-up stages of these generators, and good air circulation is necessary to eliminate it.

2. In a curtained area, turn on the generator with the shutters closed, to allow a 5-minute warm-up period. The length of the warm-up period must be increased as the generator ages.
3. Provide goggles for both the patient and the operator. Instruct the patient to keep eyes closed during the treatment, in addition to wearing the goggles.
4. Wash the area prior to exposure. The part to be treated should be free of all dirt, oil, makeup, or exudate.
5. The part is treated unclothed but should remain covered until the actual exposure commences.

Instructions for the MED Test Using the Hot Quartz Generator

Prior to any exposure, a minimal erythemal dose (MED) test should be performed to determine the appropriate exposure for a particular patient. The MED is the shortest dose that produces an erythema that appears within 1 to 6 hours and disappears within 24 hours. Each lamp has an MED associated with that particular lamp that is based on the average MED for a large number of people with a variety of skin types. Each patient must be treated based on his skin type and coloration, however, so an MED test should be run on every patient prior to initiating treatment.

1. Fashion a test strip as follows:
   a. Cut a piece of paper, cotton, or vinyl fabric about 6 × 10 in. (15 × 25 cm).
   b. Cut six holes about 0.5 in. (1 cm) in diameter in different shapes that run lengthwise, in the middle (Figure 7–1).
2. Instruct the patient regarding what you are going to do, what to expect from treatment, and what you expect of him.
3. Select an area of skin that has not been previously exposed to ultraviolet radiation (e.g., the chest or the lower abdomen). Have the patient remove all clothing and jewelry from the area selected. Wash the area with soap and water, and dry it.
4. Position the patient appropriately, without pillows, and drape completely except for the area to be exposed.
5. Attach the MED test strip to the selected area of the patient's skin. Make sure the strip is completely flat to avoid casting shadows on the exposure surface. Cover the strip with a towel.
6. Position the generator directly over the area, parallel to the surface, and 30 in. (76 cm) away. Measure perpendicularly from the actual source of the waves to the highest point on the exposed area (see Appendix B, Cosine Law).
7. Following the exposure guide below, expose the first hole, open the shutters, and begin timing immediately, using a stopwatch. The times suggested here are based on a lamp with an average MED of 30 seconds. If a patient is particularly fair, or verbally reports that he sunburns readily, the time should be shortened. Conversely, if the patient has a dark complexion and rarely burns, the time may be lengthened. The practitioner may not be able to determine the MED for patients with very dark skin. Erythema is rarely visible, and these patients rarely burn.

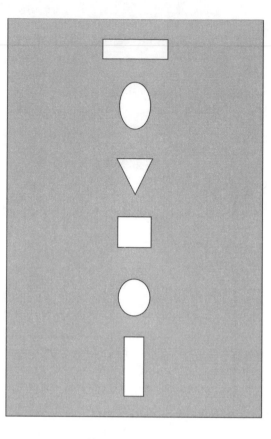

Figure 7-1. Ultraviolet test strip.

    a. First hole—30 seconds.
    b. Second hole—30 seconds.
    c. Third hole—15 seconds.
    d. Fourth hole—15 seconds.
    e. Fifth hole—15 seconds.
    f. Sixth hole—15 seconds.

8. In this way, the first hole will have received 120 seconds and the last hole 15 seconds exposure. When uncovering the holes, be sure to avoid prolonged exposure of your arm by stepping away from the lamp.

9. Close the shutters, and turn the lamp away from the patient. Leave the lamp on if it is to be used again soon. Otherwise, turn it off.

10. Allow the patient to dress.

11. Tell the patient to check the area in bright light every 2 hours while awake and to observe and record which symbols have appeared and which have faded at the time checked. Provide a form for this purpose (Figure 7–2).

12. Have the patient return the form to you at the next treatment. Determine the patient's minimal erythemal dose. Remember, the MED is the shortest dose to appear within 1 to 6 hours and to disappear within 24 hours. In Figure 7–3, the MED is 30 seconds. If all doses appear and remain longer than 24 hours, the MED has not been determined. Repeat the test with shorter doses. If no doses appear, repeat the test using longer doses.

Patient Name:	Practitioner Name:
Date:	Time of Test:
Lamp:	Skin-Source Distance:
Test Site:	MED:

Elapsed Time in Hours	Symbol					
Exposure Time in Seconds	15	30	45	60	90	120
1						
2						
4						
6						
8						
10						
12						
14						
16						
18						
20						
22						
24						

Instructions:

Begin observing the area 1 hour after exposure. Each time you check the area, make an "X" in the appropriate box for those symbols which are visible. For example, at 1 hour, the rectangle marked 120 may be visible but no others. Mark an "X" in the box under that symbol in the 1 hour row. If the rectangle remains visible for 24 hours, its column will be filled with "Xs". On the other hand, the rectangle marked 15 may never become visible and should not have any "Xs" in its column. If you were sleeping at the checking time, mark the box with an "S". When a symbol is no longer visible, discontinue marking its column.

Figure 7–2. Patient recording form for MED test.

Instructions for General Exposure: Four-Quadrant Method

1. Instruct the patient regarding what you are going to do, what to expect from treatment, and what you expect of him.
2. Turn the machine on to warm it up.
3. Position the patient supine with no pillows. The patient should be nude with protective covering over the nipples, genitalia, and eyes. The head may be turned to one side and the upper extremities placed in anatomical position.
4. Drape the patient completely, using two sheets. One sheet should cover the superior half of the body and the other, the inferior half. The edges of the two sheets should meet exactly. Tuck the sheets in so that they do not shift.
5. Center the burner directly over the superior half of the patient's body at the same distance as that used for testing. If 30 in. (76 cm) from the highest point was the distance used for testing, the same distance should be used for treatment.

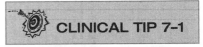

CLINICAL TIP 7–1

Draping for Ultraviolet Treatments

When draping patients for treatment with ultraviolet radiation, be sure to establish landmarks that will be reproducible on subsequent treatments. Because the dosage time increases with each treatment, any area of intact skin that has not been previously exposed could receive a serious burn.

Patient Name: XYZ	Practitioner Name: QRS
Date: 3/29/98	Time of Test: 2:00 PM
Lamp: Hot quartz	Skin-Source Distance: 30 in
Test Site: Abdomen	MED: 30 sec

Elapsed Time in Hours	Symbol					
Exposure Time in Seconds	15	30	45	60	90	120
1					X	X
2				X	X	X
4		X	X	X	X	X
6		X	X	X	X	X
8		X	X	X	X	X
10		S	S	S	S	S
12		S	S	S	S	S
14		S	S	S	S	S
16		S	S	S	S	S
18			X	X	X	X
20		X	X	X	X	X
22				X	X	X
24				X	X	X

Instructions:

Begin observing the area 1 hour after exposure. Each time you check the area, make an "X" in the appropriate box for those symbols which are visible. For example, at 1 hour, the rectangle marked 120 may be visible but no others. Mark an "X" in the box under that symbol in the 1 hour row. If the rectangle remains visible for 24 hours, its column will be filled with "Xs". On the other hand, the rectangle marked 15 may never become visible and should not have any "Xs" in its column. If you were sleeping at the checking time, mark the box with an "S". When a symbol is no longer visible, discontinue marking its column.

Figure 7–3. Completed patient recording form for MED test indicating the MED for that patient.

6. Remove the superiorly placed sheet, being sure not to move the other one. Open the shutters and time a minimal erythemal dose based on the patient's MED test.

7. Close the shutters and replace the sheet exactly as it was prior to the exposure. Move the lamp to the inferior half of the patient's body and check the skin–source distance. Remove the lower sheet, uncovering the patient to the same level as used for the superior quadrant. Make sure that no area receives double exposure but that all areas are exposed once.

8. Open the shutters and time another MED.

9. Close the shutters and replace the sheet.

10. Have the patient turn prone, with no pillows, and drape in the same manner. Be sure that the patient's head remains turned to the same side and that the upper extremities remain in anatomical position.

11. Center the lamp over the inferior half of the patient's body, check the distance, and remove the lower sheet.

12. Open the shutters, time another MED, close the shutters, and replace the sheet.

13. Move the lamp to the superior portion of the patient's body, check the skin–source distance, and remove the upper sheet. Make sure no area receives double exposure.

14. Open the shutters, time another MED, close the shutters, and replace the drape.
15. Remove the lamp and turn it off if it is not to be used again.
16. Allow the patient to dress.
17. Document the patient's responses to the previous treatment, the lamp used, lamp distance, and exposure time.

An alternative method involves covering the patient's face during the four-quadrant exposure and giving a separate minimal erythemal dose to the face while the patient is supine. The position of the head depends on where any lesions may be. If there are none, exposures to the two sides allow more even absorption.

Instructions for Local Exposure With the Hot Quartz Generator

The hot quartz generator may be used to deliver local treatment. The area to be treated is draped so that no other area is exposed, and an appropriate exposure is given following the principles described for general treatment.

Instructions for Local Exposures With the Cold Quartz Generator

The cold quartz generator is designed to be used for local treatment.

1. Instruct the patient regarding what you are going to do, what to expect from treatment, and what you expect of him.
2. Wash the area to be treated with soap and water, and clean any wounds of debris and medication. Dry the area thoroughly.
3. Position and drape the patient appropriately and provide goggles. If there is an open wound, the use of sterile drapes may be necessary.
4. Cover the generator and allow a 1- to 3-minute warm-up period, if necessary. (Some generators require no warm-up period.)
5. Position the lamp so that the waves are perpendicular to the skin surface, and ensure a 1-inch (2.5 cm) distance by propping the lamp securely with pillows or a gauze doughnut.
6. At the conclusion of the treatment, turn off the generator and give appropriate follow-up care.
7. Document patient response to the previous treatment, lamp used, lamp distance, and exposure time.

DOSAGE

Intensity and Time for the Hot Quartz Generator

Dosage depends on the condition—specifically, whether the skin is intact. Generally, mucosal surfaces can tolerate twice as much ultraviolet radiation from any source as epidermal tissues. Healing wounds may be treated with MED or E_1 doses from any UVB or UVC source. Indolent ulcers or infected wounds may be treated with E_2 or E_3 doses from any UVB or UVC source to stimulate repair, destroy bacteria, and increase blood supply.

The intensity of the reaction to ultraviolet radiation is based on time of exposure. Therefore, dosage is based on the time needed to produce the desired effects. The doses used with hot quartz generators set at 30 in. (76 cm) are summarized in Table 7–2. For small areas, shorter distances may be used, but the dosage time should be recalculated by the formula given below. Never use a hot quartz generator at distances less than 15 in. (38 cm). The operating temperature is high enough that the patient could receive a thermal burn.

$$T_2 = \frac{T_1 d_2{}^2}{d_1{}^2}$$

where

T_1 = Initial time
T_2 = New time
d_1 = Initial distance
d_2 = New distance

Intensity and Time for the Cold Quartz Generator

If the cold quartz generator is used for mucosal tissue, an MED test is not necessary. For treatment of intact skin an MED test should be performed. Table 7–3 may be used as a guide to dosage for treatment of mucosal tissues with the cold quartz generator or if performing an MED test is not feasible.

Progression

Due to the thickening of the epidermis and the deposition of melanin, MED exposures to intact skin should be increased by 25% with each treatment to maintain the same level of response. An E_1 dose can be increased by 50%, and an E_2 dose can be increased by 75% of the preceding dose.[19] Doses to mucosal tissue need not be increased because of the lack of epidermal covering. For every missed treatment, decrease the next exposure by 25% of the previous dose. After a period without treatment, or following desquamation, a return to the initial dose is indicated.

Frequency

No dose of ultraviolet radiation should be repeated until the erythema produced by the previous dose has disappeared. An MED can be repeated daily,

TABLE 7–2. Doses Used With Hot Quartz Generators of Ultraviolet Radiation

DOSE	DESCRIPTION	RELATIONSHIP TO MED	USE
Suberythemal dose (SED)	Produces no erythema but can produce vitamin D		Appropriate for full body exposure
Minimal erythemal dose (MED)	The *smallest* dose producing *any* erythema that appears in 1 to 6 hours and that fades without a trace within 24 hours		Appropriate for total body exposures or local treatments
First-degree erythemal dose (E_1)	Produces erythema that lasts for 1 to 3 days with clear reddening and some mild desquamation	2.5 times the MED[19]	Should be given only to areas of less than 20% of body surface[19]
Second-degree erythemal dose (E_2)	Produces intense erythema with edema, peeling, and pigmentation	5 times the MED[19]	Should be given only to areas less than 250 cm² in area[19]
Third-degree erythemal dose (E_3)	Produces erythema with severe blistering, peeling, and exudation	10 times the MED[19]	Should be given only to areas less than 25 cm² in area[19]

TABLE 7–3. Dosages for Cold Quartz Treatment

DOSE	DISTANCE (INCHES)	EXPOSURE (SECONDS)
MED	1	12–15
E_1	1	30–45
E_2	1	72–90
E_3	1	135–180

Adapted from Birtcher Corporation "Spot Quartz" Instruction Manual; 1962.

because the erythema, by definition, must have disappeared within 24 hours. An E_1 dose is repeated approximately on alternate days, whereas an E_2 dose is repeated in three to four days. Treatments to mucosal surfaces may be repeated daily.[19]

RESPONSES TO TREATMENT AND TREATMENT MODIFICATION

Depending on the condition, normal responses range from a slight reddening of the skin to peeling of the epidermis. A patient with dark skin does not demonstrate an erythema unless the dose is quite large.[20] Doses that produce blisters should be avoided. A patient with excessive general exposure may experience tissue damage severe enough to produce symptoms of protein shock such as pallor, shallow pulse, shallow respiration, and low blood pressure.[11]

HOME USE

In most cases, ultraviolet treatment is inappropriate for home use. Excessive exposure to ultraviolet radiation is hazardous. Due to the inherent severity of tissue responses, if the treatment is inadvertently given for too long or the lamp placed too close, serious burns or systemic reactions could occur. In addition, the patient should be cautioned about the risks of sunbathing without using ultraviolet-blocking skin preparations and about the potential hazards of the tanning salons that have recently become popular. These salons are unregulated, and operators may or may not have knowledge concerning the effects and hazards of ultraviolet radiation.

REFERENCES

1. McGrath H. Ultraviolet-A1 irradiation decreases clinical disease activity and autoantibodies in patients with systemic lupus erythematosus. *Clin Exp Rheumatol.* 1994; 12:129–135.
2. Daniels F. Ultraviolet light and dermatology. In: Stillwell K, ed. *Therapeutic Electricity and Ultraviolet Radiation.* 3rd ed. Baltimore: Williams & Wilkins; 1983:263–303.
3. Scott PM. *Clayton's Electrotherapy and Actinotherapy.* 7th ed. Baltimore: Williams & Wilkins; 1975.
4. Taylor GJS, Leeming JP, Bannister GC. Effect of antiseptics, ultraviolet light and lavage on airborne bacteria in a model wound. *J Bone Joint Surg.* 1993;75-B:724–730.

5. Nussbaum EL, Biemann I, Mustard B. Comparison of ultrasound/ultraviolet-C and laser for treatment of pressure ulcers in patients with spinal cord injury. *Phys Ther.* 1994;74:812–825.

6. Agency for Health Care Policy and Research. *Clinical Practice Guideline Number 15: Treatment of Pressure Ulcers.* Rockville, Md: US Department of Health and Human Services; 1994. AHCPR Publication No. 95-0652.

7. Fitch DH, Soderstrom RM, Kinzie S. PUVA therapy in the treatment of psoriasis. *Clin Manage Phys Ther.* 1987;7(4):24, 26–27.

8. Gilchrest BA, Rowe JW, Brown RS, et al. Relief of uremic pruritis with ultraviolet phototherapy. *N Engl J Med.* 1977;297:136–138.

9. Scott BO. Clinical uses of ultraviolet radiation. In: Stillwell K, ed. *Therapeutic Electricity and Ultraviolet Radiation.* 3rd ed. Baltimore: Williams & Wilkins; 1983:228–262.

10. Griffin JE, Karselis TC. *Physical Agents for Physical Therapists.* Springfield, Ill: Charles C Thomas; 1978.

11. Shriber WJ. *A Manual of Electrotherapy.* 4th ed. Philadelphia: Lea & Febiger; 1975.

12. Harber LC, Bickers DR. *Photosensitivity Diseases: Principles of Diagnosis and Treatment.* 2nd ed. Toronto: B.C. Decker; 1989.

13. Cohen MR, Isenberg DA. Ultraviolet irradiation in systemic lupus erythematosus: friend or foe? *Br J Rheumatol.* 1996;35:1002–1007.

14. McGrath H, Martinez-Osuna P, Lee FA. Ultraviolet-A1 (340–400 nm) irradiation therapy in systemic lupus erythematosus. *Lupus.* 1996;5:269–274.

15. Molina JF, McGrath J. Longterm ultraviolet-A1 irradiation therapy in systemic lupus erythematosus. *J Rheumatol.* 1997;24:1072–1074.

16. *Physician's Desk Reference.* 52nd ed. Oradell, NJ: Medical Economics Company; 1998.

17. Montgomery PC. The compounding effects of infrared and ultraviolet irradiation upon normal human skin. *Phys Ther.* 1973;53:489–496.

18. Diffey BL. Ultraviolet radiation and skin cancer. *Physiotherapy.* 1989;75:615–616.

19. Wadsworth H, Chanmugan APP. *Electrophysical Agents in Physiotherapy: Therapeutic and Diagnostic Use.* 2nd. ed. Marrickville, NSW, Australia: Science Press; 1983.

20. Diffey BL, Robson J. The influence of pigmentation and illumination on the perception of erythema. *Photodermatol Photoimmunol Photomed.* 1992;9:45–47.

ADDITIONAL READINGS

Basford JR, Hallman HO, Sheffield CG, Mackey GL. Comparison of cold-quartz ultraviolet, low-energy laser, and occlusion in wound healing in a swine model. *Arch Phys Med Rehabil.* 1986;67:151–154.

Fenske NA. How the sun aggravates age-related skin changes. *Mod Med.* 1982;50(12):147–154.

Fusco RJ, Jordan PA, Kelly A, Samuel M. PUVA treatment for psoriasis. *Physiotherapy.* 1980;66:39–40.

Goats GC. Appropriate use of the inverse square law. *Physiotherapy.* 1988;74:8.

Gorham H. Treatment of psoriatic arthropathy by PUVA. *Physiotherapy.* 1980;66:40.

Klaber MR. Ultra-violet light for psoriasis. *Physiotherapy.* 1980;66:36–38.

Kloth LC. Physical modalities in wound management: UVC, therapeutic heating and electrical stimulation. *Ostomy/Wound Manage.* 1995;41:18–27.

Low J. Quantifying the erythema due to UVR. *Physiotherapy.* 1986;72:60–64.

Shurr DG, Zuehlke RL. Photochemotherapy treatment for psoriasis. *Phys Ther.* 1981;61:33–36.

Solomon WM, Netherton EW, Nelson PA, Zeiter WJ. Treatment of psoriasis with the Goeckerman technique. *Arch Phys Med Rehabil.* 1955;36:74–77.

Taylor RB. Clinical study of ultraviolet in various skin conditions. *Phys Ther.* 1972;52:279–282.

Tromovitch TA, Thompson LR, Jacobs PH. Testing for photosensitivity. *J Am Phys Ther Assoc.* 1963;43:348–349.

Van Scott EJ. Therapy of psoriasis 1975. *JAMA.* 1976;235:197.

8

Intermittent Compression Pump

DESCRIPTION

Compression pumps are pneumatic units designed to apply external pressure to an edematous body part. The apparatus consists of a two-layered nylon or plastic appliance shaped to fit either the upper or lower extremity. Pressure is provided by air that is pumped between the two layers via rubber tubing. The amount of pressure and the time for which it is applied are adjustable. Appliances may have single or multiple compartments with separate tubes and controls (Figures 8–1 and 8–2). These compartments can be filled sequentially and, in some cases, to different pressures.

PURPOSE AND EFFECTS

External pressure, when applied to an edematous extremity, helps reduce edema by moving excess interstitial fluid to sites of normal lymphatic or venous drainage. The pressure should be higher distally and lower proximally to approximate normal hydrostatic pressure and move the fluid proximally. External compression has also been found to decrease pain and improve range of motion, presumably secondarily to decreasing swelling.[1] There is little effect on blood flow with the use of compression[2]; some users have shown that there may be a decrease in blood flow secondary to the temporary increase in peripheral resistance.[3] There is also some concern that there may be a rebound increase in blood flow once the garment has been removed.[4]

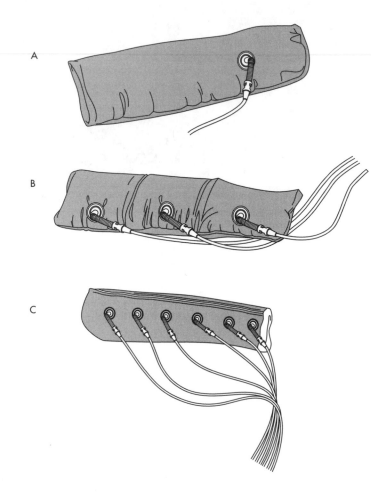

Figure 8–1. A. Single compartment compression appliance. B and C. Multiple compartment appliances for the upper extremity.

INDICATIONS

1. Postmastectomy lymphedema.[5,6] Open the lymphatic channels using manual lymphatic massage prior to using the pump.[7]
2. Traumatic edema.[1,8]
3. Dependent edema of pregnancy.[9,10]
4. Venous insufficiency.[11]
5. Amputations.[12]
6. Prevention of thrombophlebitis postsurgically.[13]
7. Stasis ulcers.[14]

CONTRAINDICATIONS

1. Patients with arterial insufficiency have increased peripheral resistance, and compression increases it further.
2. Infections at the site of treatment may be spread by introducing bacteria into the lymphatic or venous drainage.

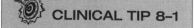

CLINICAL TIP 8–1

Using Manual Drainage With Intermittent Compression

Prepare the trunk with manual lymphatic drainage (massage) prior to the use of the compression pump.

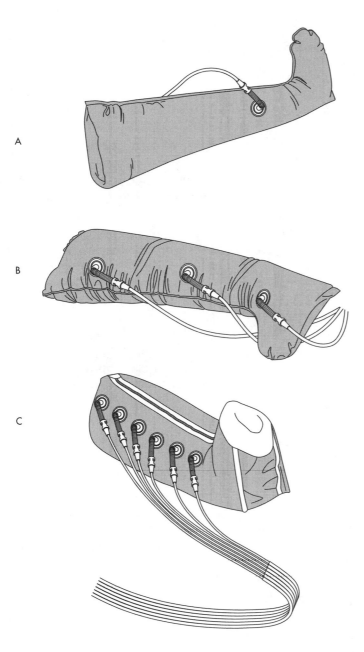

Figure 8-2. A. Single compartment compression appliance. B and C. Multiple compartment compression appliances for the lower extremity.

3. Any thrombi present may become mobile.
4. Edema in patients with congestive heart failure should not be treated, because the increased peripheral resistance increases the work of the heart.
5. Edema in patients with kidney dysfunction should not be treated, because the kidney may not be able to excrete the additional fluid.
6. Obstructed lymphatic channels do not allow drainage. Treatment is ineffective, and the patient may experience increased pain.
7. Displaced fractures. Treatment may displace them further.

INSTRUCTIONS

1. Instruct the patient regarding the treatment and what you expect of her.
2. Check the patient's skin integrity and pressure sensation, and measure the girth of the part to be treated. Determine the patient's blood pressure.
3. Position the patient comfortably with the part to be treated at about 30 degrees of elevation.
4. Apply stockinette to the extremity, covering it entirely. Make sure it is smooth. A rigid finger or toe protector may be fashioned to prevent excessive compression of the digits.[15]
5. Apply the appliance and attach the rubber tubing.
6. To inflate the appliance, set the unit to apply pressure continually while the exhaust cycle is off.
7. Increase the pressure to the patient's tolerance without exceeding the diastolic blood pressure. The patient should feel *no* pain, tingling, numbness, or pulse during treatment.
8. Once the pressure is adjusted, reset the unit to cycle. The cycle can and should be varied according to the patient's tolerance. Units that have multiple, sequentially filling compartments fill the distal compartment first.
9. During the exhaust cycle, encourage the patient to exercise her fingers or toes.
10. The minimum treatment should be 2 hours out of every 24 hours. More effective reduction of edema is achieved if the patient is treated for 2 hours twice daily. However, decreases have been achieved in less time. Positive results have been achieved in some patients with lymphedema with 30-minute sessions, three times a week.[16]
11. Remove the appliance hourly to check the skin and allow some exercise.
12. At the conclusion of treatment, remove the appliance and perform all appropriate posttreatment evaluation procedures, including skin inspection, blood pressure, and girth measurements.
13. To retain the reduction, wrap the part with an elastic bandage and instruct the patient in its use and application. Low-stretch bandages are recommended for patients with lymphedema.[7]
14. Document patient position, extremity preparation, appliance used, pressures used, duration of treatment, and all patient responses.

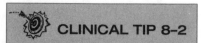

CLINICAL TIP 8-2

Treatment Combination With Intermittent Compression

The effect of intermittent pneumatic compression is enhanced if is it coupled with elevation of the extremity. Treatment effects may also be intensified if compression is combined with cold treatments and muscle pumping exercises.

RESPONSES TO TREATMENT AND TREATMENT MODIFICATION

The patient should experience only a sense of pressure during the treatment and feel *no* pain, tingling, numbness, or pulse from the pressure. If the patient does experience any of these sensations, reduce the pressure. Following treatment a reduction of swelling should result. There may be some skin indentations if there were wrinkles in the skin covering. As the patient tolerates the treatment, "on" times, "off" times and total treatment time may be increased with subsequent treatments.

DOSAGE

Intensity

The pressure should be set to the patient's tolerance without exceeding the diastolic blood pressure. Generally, keeping pressures at less than 50 mm for the upper extremity and 60 mm for the lower extremity should be safe and effective.[17] When treating lymphedema, a maximum pressure of 45 mm Hg is recommended.[18] For units with multiple compartments and separate pressure controls, the difference between compartmental pressures may be about 20 mm, with the distal compartment having the highest pressure.[15]

Once the pressure is adjusted, adjust the cycling so that pressure is applied for about 45 to 90 seconds and released for about 15 to 30 seconds. Usually, the pressure is applied in a 3:1 ratio of pressure to exhaust according to the patient's tolerance. Units that have multiple, sequentially filling compartments fill the distal compartment first. The more proximal compartments inflate at 20 second intervals.[15] In some equipment, the cycle time is preset by the manufacturer.

Duration

The minimum treatment should be 2 hours out of every 24 hours. More effective reduction of edema is achieved if the patient is treated for 2 hours twice daily, although some practitioners obtain success using a single session daily, three days per week.[16]

Frequency

The pump should be used daily or twice daily until maximum reduction of edema is achieved, in approximately 3 to 4 weeks. Girth measurements, before and after treatment, should be performed until no further change is detected. A compression garment should then be fitted to maintain the reduction if the condition is chronic.

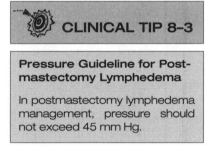

CLINICAL TIP 8-3

Pressure Guideline for Postmastectomy Lymphedema

In postmastectomy lymphedema management, pressure should not exceed 45 mm Hg.

HOME USE

Due to the long treatment time, rental of a unit for home use should be considered. Be sure to instruct the patient regarding positioning, extremity preparation, amount of pressure, cycling, and duration and frequency.

REFERENCES

1. Airaksinen O. Changes in posttraumatic ankle joint mobility, pain, and edema following intermittent pneumatic compression therapy. *Arch Phys Med Rehabil.* 1989; 70:341–344.
2. Rucinski TJ, Hooker DN, Prentice WE, et al. The effects of intermittent compression on edema in postacute ankle sprains. *J Orthop Sports Phys Ther.* 1991;14:65–69.
3. Rithalia SVS, Edwards J, Sayegh A. Effect of intermittent pneumatic compression on lower limb oxygenation. *Arch Phys Med Rehabil.* 1988; 69:665–667.
4. Quillen WS, Rouillier LH. Initial management of acute ankle sprains with rapid pulsed pneumatic compression and cold. *J Orthop Sports Phys Ther.* 1982;4:39–43.

5. Swedborg I. Effects of treatment with an elastic sleeve and intermittent pneumatic compression in post-mastectomy patients with lymphoedema of the arm. *Scand J Rehabil Med.* 1984;16:35–41.
6. Mridha M, Ödman S. Fluid translocation measurement. *Scand J Rehabil Med.* 1989; 21:63–69.
7. Reul-Hirche H. Physiotherapy management of lymphedema. In: Sapsford R, Bullock-Saxton J, Markwell S, eds. *Women's Health: A Textbook for Physiotherapists.* London: W. B. Saunders; 1998.
8. Airaksinen O, Kolari PJ, Herve R, Holopainen R. Treatment of post-traumatic oedema in lower legs using intermittent pneumatic compression. *Scand J Rehabil Med.* 1988; 20:25–28.
9. Jacobs MK, McCance KL, Stewart ML. External pneumatic intermittent compression for treatment of dependent pregnancy edema. *Nurs Res.* 1982;31:159–162, 191.
10. Jacobs MK, McCance KL, Stewart ML. Leg volume changes with EPIC and posturing in dependent pregnancy edema. *Nurs Res.* 1986;35:86–89.
11. Sussman C, Bates-Jensen BM. *Wound Care.* Gaithersburg, Md: Aspen Publishers; 1998.
12. Condie E, Treweek S, Jones D, Scott H. A one-year national survey of patients having a lower limb amputation. *Physiotherapy.* 1996;82:14–20.
13. Clark WB, MacGregor AB, Prescott RJ, Ruckley CV. Pneumatic compression of the calf and postoperative deep-vein thrombosis. *Lancet.* 1974;1(7871):5–6.
14. McCulloch JM. Intermittent compression for the treatment of a chronic stasis ulceration: a case report. *Phys Ther.* 1981;61:1452–1453.
15. Klein MJ, Alexander MA, Wright JM, et al. Treatment of adult lower extremity lymphedema with the Wright linear pump: statistical analysis of a clinical trial. *Arch Phys Med Rehabil.* 1988;69:202–206.
16. Tipton JP, Barsotti J, Gaisne E, Vaillant L. A survey of the French-speaking Association of Lymphology on the use of pressotherapy in France during the treatment of lymphedema. *J Mal Vasc.* 1990;15:270–276.
17. Beninson J. Lymphedema: patho-physiologic and clinical concepts. *Angiology.* 1975; 26:661–664.
18. Casley-Smith J, Casley-Smith JR. Aetiologies of lymphoedema. In: Casley-Smith J, Casley-Smith JR, eds. *Modern Treatment for Lymphoedema.* Adelaide, Australia: The Lymphoedema Association of Australia; 1994.

ADDITIONAL READINGS

Dervin GF, Taylor DE, Keene GCR. Effects of cold and compression dressings on early postoperative outcomes for the arthroscopic anterior cruciate ligament reconstruction patient. *J Orthop Sports Phys Ther.* 1998;27:403–406.

Griffin JW, Newsome LS, Stralka SW, Wright PE. Reduction of chronic posttraumatic hand edema: a comparison of high voltage pulsed current, intermittent pneumatic compression, and placebo treatments. *Phys Ther.* 1990;70:279–286.

Hartmann BR, Drews B, Kayser T. Physical therapy improves venous hemodynamics in cases of primary varicosity: results of a controlled study. *Angiology.* 1997;48:157–162.

Jungi WF. The prevention and management of lymphoedema after treatment for breast cancer. *Int Rehabil Med.* 1981;3:129–134.

Kolb P, Denegar C. Traumatic edema and the lymphatic system. *Athletic Training.* 1983;17: 339–341.

Matsen FA, Krugmire RB. The effect of externally applied pressure on post-fracture swelling. *J Bone Joint Surg.* 1974;56-A:1586–1591.

Murphy K. The combination of ice and intermittent compression system in the treatment of soft tissue injuries. *Physiotherapy.* 1988;74:41.

Nelson PA. Recent advances in treatment of lymphedema of the extremities. *Geriatrics.* 1966;21:162–173.

Sanderson RG, Fletcher WS. Conservative management of primary lymphedema. *Northwest Med.* 1965;64:584–588.

Swedborg I. Voluminometric estimation of the degree of lymphedema and its therapy by pneumatic compression. *Scand J Rehabil Med.* 1977;9:131–135.

Wilkerson J. Contrast baths and pressure treatment for ankle sprains. *Physician Sportsmed.* 1979;7:143.

Mechanical Spinal Traction

Jane Wilding

DESCRIPTION

Mechanical spinal traction involves the use of electronic traction units that exert a pulling force through a rope and various halters and straps. The tractive force results in a longitudinal separation and gliding apart of cervical or lumbar spinal segments.

PURPOSE AND EFFECTS

The main purpose of mechanical traction is to reduce signs or symptoms of cervical or lumbar spinal compression. There are several mechanisms by which symptom reduction is accomplished.

1. Gently stretching facet joint capsules. The direction of gliding depends on the angle of pull and the position of the spinal segments.[1]
2. Increasing the inferior-superior dimensions of the intervertebral foramina, allowing increased space for spinal nerve roots.[2–6]
3. Elongating posterior muscle tissue, decreasing its sensitivity to stretch and decreasing muscle guarding.[7]
4. Improving blood supply to the posterior soft tissues and the intervertebral discs. Traction decreases the intradiscal pressure, and osmosis from the vertebral endplates brings increased blood supply to the disc.[8–10]
5. Altering intradiscal pressure. Decreasing the positive pressure may reduce a bulging of the nuclear material.[9,11,12]

INDICATIONS

Medical diagnoses that may be suitable for treatment using mechanical traction include low back or neck pain, degenerative disc disease, osteoarthritis, spondylosis, herniated nucleus pulposus, foraminal stenosis, apophyseal joint impingement, and muscle spasm.

1. Spinal nerve root impingement due to degenerative disc disease (bulging, herniation, protrusion). Vertebral separation helps decrease intradiscal pressure (if not sustained beyond 10 minutes) and increase the superior-inferior dimension of the intervertebral foramen. Tightening the annular fibers and the posterior longitudinal ligament can flatten a bulge.
2. Spinal nerve root impingement due to spinal stenosis. Vertebral body separation, typically in a relative forward-bending direction, increases the superior-inferior dimension of the intervertebral foramen and possibly relieves nerve root impingement resulting from narrowing.
3. Generalized hypomobility of lumbar or cervical spine regions. Longitudinal traction force provides a gliding separation of facets, general capsular stretch, and opening of the intervertebral foramen.
4. Muscle spasm resulting in nerve root impingement at the intervertebral foramen or aggravation of facet or disc signs, symptoms, or both. Usually, gentle, intermittent traction assists in decreasing the muscle spasm and the resultant compression.

    If patient examinations reveal one or more of the following signs and symptoms, the patient's condition may be appropriate for an intervention plan incorporating mechanical traction.
5. Musculoskeletal signs.
    a. Positive neurologic signs such as decreased sensation, motor function, or reflexes that are temporarily improved by manual traction.
    b. General hypomobility of the spine.
    c. Local spinal hypomobility and associated increased muscle tone that reduces with manual or positional traction.
6. Musculoskeletal symptoms.
    a. Extremity numbness, pain, or tingling that is temporarily relieved by manual or positional traction.
    b. Central, unilateral, or bilateral spinal pain reduced by manual or positional traction.

CONTRAINDICATIONS

Absolute

1. Spinal infections (e.g., meningitis, arachnoiditis). Infection could be spread through the use of traction.
2. Spinal cancer. Mechanical traction may increase the danger of metastases or promote instability. Manual traction may be used for symptom reduction.
3. Spinal cord pressure. If the patient is exhibiting bilateral neurologic signs, a serious pathology such as a large disc prolapse, tumor, or severe osteophytes may be indicated. Traction may aggravate the condition.

4. Rheumatoid arthritis. Joint capsules, ligaments, and bones are fragile. Patients are subject to atlantoaxial subluxation or to developing instability next to areas of hypomobility.
5. Osteoporosis. Bones are fragile and subject to fracture.
6. Recent fracture. Bones are unstable and may be misaligned from the movement.
7. For lumbar traction, any condition that is likely to be aggravated from increased abdominal pressure produced by the corsets used in lumbar traction. This includes abdominal or hiatal hernia, uncontrolled hypertension, aortic aneurysm, and severe hemorrhoids.

Relative

1. Ligamentous strains and joint hypermobility. If manual testing or active range of motion indicates ligamentous strain or increased mobility of particular segments, traction should not incorporate these segments. Common areas include the atlantoaxial, cervicothoracic, thoracolumbar, and lumbosacral junctions. Manual traction may be used to improve segment specificity.
2. Acute stages of injury. Inflammation may be adding mechanical pressure to joint structures via swelling. The traction force may aggravate the inflammation.
3. "Traction anxiety." If the patient cannot relax or is very anxious about trying traction, use manual traction first to teach the patient how to release muscles gradually in a supportive environment. In some cases, the patient's negative perception prohibits the use of mechanical traction.
4. Cardiac or respiratory insufficiency. Monitor the patient's pulse rate, blood pressure, and respiratory functions. If the traction harness or anxiety produces negative changes in vital signs, use manual traction.
5. Pregnancy. Pregnant women have increased ligamentous laxity, and ligaments should not be stretched further. Because of the pressure, the pelvic harness cannot be used. Cervical traction may be done with caution, but manual traction is the method of choice.

INSTRUCTIONS

1. Instruct the patient regarding what to expect and what you expect of him. Patient understanding, comfort, safety, and cooperation are vital to successful outcomes. Explain the patient's role by giving a brief explanation of how the traction unit works, how it is intended to affect the individual's specific signs and symptoms, and how it should feel. Instruct the patient to relax as much as possible. Tell the patient to report any increase in symptoms or discomfort from the equipment.
2. Position the patient in an appropriate, comfortable position. A position that encourages maximum patient relaxation is desired. In general, position the segment or segments to be treated about midway between flexion and extension (i.e., loose pack position), determining the specific angle by manual traction and palpation.

Cervical Traction

For cervical treatments, either the supine or sitting position may be used. The supine position provides improved muscle relaxation, vertebral separation, and easier countertraction.[13] If the supine position is used, place a pillow under the patient's knees. If the sitting position is used, support the patient through the lower extremities, pelvic girdle, lumbar and thoracic spine, and upper extremities.

If the segment to be treated is below C-2, position the cervical spine in 20 to 30 degrees of flexion,[14] just sufficient to flatten the lordosis. Flexing beyond this neutral position for the segment decreases the intervertebral space as the ligamentum flavum tightens. If the atlantoaxial segment is treated, allow the normal lordosis to remain and treat the patient in neutral (0 degrees of flexion).

Lumbar Traction

For lumbar treatments, either the supine (Figure 9–1) or prone (Figure 9–2) position may be used. The supine, hooklying position is appropriate for general facet hypomobility, intervertebral joint hypomobility, or stenosis. Varying degrees of flexion allow increased facet and intervertebral foramen separation. The prone, neutral spine position may be more appropriate for disc conditions, especially if posterior or posterolateral bulging or protrusion is present. A flexed position produces increased anterior loading and resultant posterior bulging. A neutral to extended position increases posterior loading and resultant anterior movement of nuclear material. Raising or lowering the height of the traction table alters the rope angle to the table. This affects the degree of flexion or extension pull on the lumbar segments.

3. Apply the appropriate halter or corsets.

Cervical Traction

For cervical treatment, apply the head halter under the mandible and on the occiput and attach it to the spreader bar (Figure 9–3). The rope must be slack to attach the spreader bar, but the slack should be removed prior

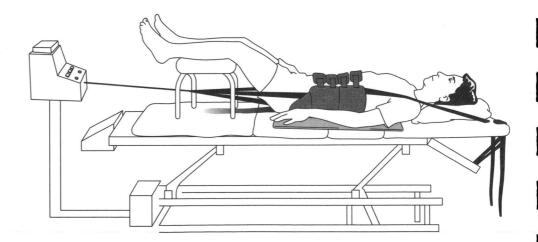

Figure 9–1. Lumbar traction in the supine position.

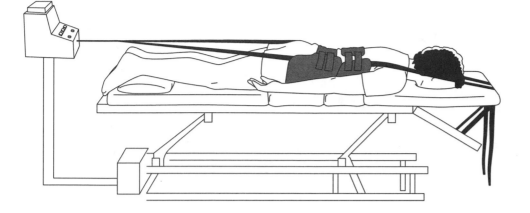

Figure 9–2. Lumbar traction in the prone position.

to initiating treatment. Adjust the halter so that the pull is absorbed mostly by the occiput. If the line of pull is set too anteriorly to the posterior neck structures, the traction pulls the neck into extension. If the head halter crosses the temporomandibular joint, irritation of the joint complex may occur. An occipital harness can be used in place of a halter. The occipital harness consists of a padded occipital headrest and a forehead strap that are pulled on a track connected to the machine (Figure 9–4). The harness is effective in eliminating temporomandibular joint pressure.

Lumbar Traction

For lumbar treatment, both a pelvic and a thoracic harness are used. Traction is applied to the lumbar spine through the pelvic harness, and the thoracic harness provides countertraction. Both harnesses should be worn against the skin to prevent slipping. The pelvic harness should be positioned so that its superior margin lies just above the iliac crests. Position the thoracic harness snugly around the inferior rim of ribs 8, 9,

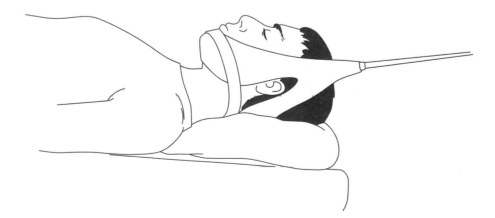

Figure 9–3. Cloth cervical traction harness.

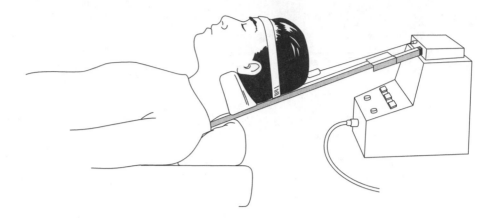

Figure 9–4. Sliding track harness for cervical traction.

and 10 and below the breasts. The bottom margin of the thoracic harness should overlap with the top margin of the pelvic belt (Figure 9–5). Secure the suspender straps of the thoracic harness to the head end of the table. The straps from the pelvic harness should be connected to the rope that provides the tractive force. Tighten both of the harnesses so

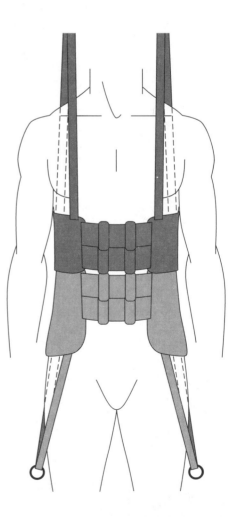

Figure 9–5. Adjustment of thoracic and pelvic harnesses for lumbar traction.

that they fit snugly and do not slip. Adjust the straps to produce the desired line of pull.

4. Decide whether to give the traction bilaterally or unilaterally. This decision is based on the patient's presenting signs and symptoms and the desired outcome of the treatment. Traction may be given unilaterally to patients demonstrating unilateral signs and symptoms such as unilateral joint hypomobility or muscle guarding, and when symptom alleviation is greater with manual unilateral traction.

Cervical Traction

When using unilateral cervical traction, the head halter is aligned at an angle to the traction source in the frontal plane. This produces cervical lateral flexion. The cervical spine should be positioned in 20 to 30 degrees of flexion and an amount of lateral flexion appropriate to the segment being treated (Figure 9–6). A stabilization strap across the patient's chest is usually required to prevent the patient from aligning himself with the angle of the rope during the treatment.[1]

Lumbar Traction

Attach the pelvic harness to the traction unit on only the affected side (Figure 9–7). The table and traction unit may be angled to produce a greater side-bending angle. Additional stabilizing straps may be necessary to control or prevent the patient from realigning.

For protective scoliosis secondary to a herniated disc, if the patient leans away from the side of pain, the protrusion is lateral to the nerve root.[15] If the patient leans over the painful side, the protrusion is medial to the nerve root. Saunders suggests giving traction on the convex side of the curve in either case.[16] Base the decision (i.e., bilateral, left unilateral, or right unilateral) on how the patient responds best to testing with manual traction.

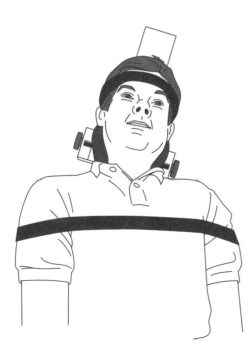

Figure 9–6. Unilateral cervical traction setup.

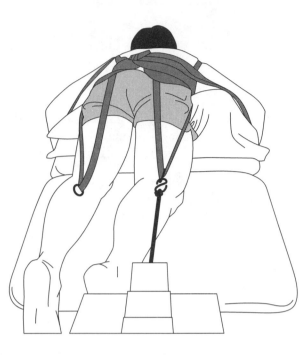

Figure 9-7. Unilateral (prone) lumbar traction setup.

5. Select the appropriate treatment mode and duration. Mechanical traction may be administered either statically (sustained) or intermittently. This decision should be made by determining the goal of treatment. To relieve a muscle that is guarding, two possible mechanisms should be considered. One involves silencing the stretch reflex, and the other involves stimulating the muscle pump to increase blood flow. Electrical silence in response to stretch occurs only after 3 minutes of sustained stretch.[17] Therefore, to silence the muscle spindle and relieve the guarding with traction, consider using low-weight sustained traction. Alternatively, cycling at a comfortable rate stimulates the stretch reflex, causing intermittent muscle contraction and increasing blood flow.[18] Studies suggest that, in terms of muscle activity, there is little or no difference between the two methods.[4,8] Intermittent traction may be associated with decreased posttraction discomfort.[19]

   If the goal of treatment is to relieve nerve root compression through separation of posterior structures, maximal separation occurs within 7 seconds.[4] Additional time produces no further separation. A balanced cycle is usually perceived as more pleasant, so 7 seconds on and 7 seconds off is appropriate.

   Some equipment provides for progressive and regressive steps of traction. These steps allow the patient to adjust gradually to the onset and release of the pull. Regressive traction over a period of 2 to 5 minutes may prove safe and effective.[20]

6. Determine the appropriate traction dosage. The goal of treatment, the force of the pull in pounds, the mode of traction used, and the duration of treatment govern dosage.

7. Give the patient the safety switch and explain that if pressed, the traction gradually decreases to zero force. Tell the patient to use the switch if he experiences discomfort, and the therapist does not respond immediately.

8. If using a split table to perform lumbar traction, unlock the traction table. Start the traction program.

9. Monitor the patient's signs and symptoms before, during, and after treatment.

10. At the conclusion of treatment, turn off the machine. Release the rope gently and gradually, making sure that no residual tension on the rope remains. If the tension is not released gradually, rebound of intradiscal pressure or a shift of cerebrospinal fluid could occur, leading to dizziness, headaches, or an increase in symptoms.

11. Remove all equipment and allow the patient to rest for at least 1 to 2 minutes before arising. If using a split table to perform lumbar traction, lock the traction table before allowing the patient to rise.

12. Perform all appropriate posttreatment examinations, including neurologic testing.

13. Adequate recording of traction parameters used in a single treatment session is essential. Without adequate documentation, it is difficult to reproduce or modify treatment in subsequent sessions or to monitor the patient's response from previous treatment sessions effectively. The information that should be recorded in the patient's medical record includes type of traction, target area, patient position, angle of pull, mode of traction, dosage, duration of treatment, and patient response.

DOSAGE

Intensity

The intensity of traction is determined by the amount of pull exerted on the patient. In general, the force reported by the patient to provide the greatest degree of comfort without negative change in neurologic status during or following the treatment should be used. If traction feels irritating to the patient, it may result in increased muscle guarding and spasm that could cause actual increase in compressive loading of the vertebral joint complex.

CERVICAL TRACTION. For cervical treatment, pull is determined by patient comfort and may be progressively increased with subsequent treatments. To achieve separation of vertebral components, at least 25 lb is necessary.[14] The usual range of treatment weight is 25 to 45 lb. However, as little as 10 lb of traction has been shown to cause separation of the atlantooccipital and atlantoaxial joints.[1] Encourage the patient to relax with the pull. If he resists, no benefit will be achieved.[21,22]

LUMBAR TRACTION. When treatment is given to the lumbar spine in the supine position, the force must be sufficient to overcome friction before intervertebral separation can be achieved. A pull of half the weight of the body part is necessary for intervertebral separation.[23,24] For lumbar treatments, a minimum force equal to 25% to 50% of the patient's body weight is necessary to overcome friction. If using a split table, friction is decreased substantially, and the initial weight may be lower. However, lumbar traction forces that are below 25% of the total body weight when using a split table can be regarded as sham *treatment* (or low dose) traction.[23-25]

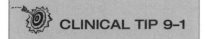

CLINICAL TIP 9–1

How to Choose the Most Effective Combination of Traction Treatment Parameters

1. First decide the therapeutic goal of the traction treatment. For example, to elicit facet joint capsular stretch, to reduce intradiscal pressure, to decrease muscle guarding, and so on.
2. Choose a patient position that allows you to meet this goal effectively. For example, if the goal were to reduce intradiscal pressure in the lumbar spine, a prone neutral spine position would be more desirable than a supine hooklying position.
3. Choose the combination of traction parameters that allows you to achieve the therapeutic goal. Many factors influence this decision, including patient comfort, pattern of pain, and healing stage. For example, to reduce facet impingement of the lumbar spine, you could choose a unilateral pull on the restricted side, with either sustained or intermittent for 10 to 15 minutes. The amount of pull would need to be more than 25% of the patient's total body weight to have any effect on the lumbar spine. If the patient's condition was not irritable, a higher weight could be chosen for the first treatment.

Time

Intermittent traction is usually performed for 20 to 30 minutes. Sustained traction is done for 3 to 30 minutes at low weights. For discogenic pain, use either sustained traction for no longer than 10 minutes or intermittent traction with a cycle of 60 seconds on and 20 seconds off for 10 to 15 minutes. Longer or shorter times may be indicated by changes in signs and symptoms. If the treatment is too long, intradiscal pressure may increase from imbibition of too much fluid, and symptoms may be aggravated following treatment.

Frequency

Frequency depends on the patient's response. Traction may be done daily, twice daily, or two to three times a week.

RESPONSES TO TREATMENT AND TREATMENT MODIFICATION

Decreased pain with decreased neurologic signs usually are an indication that the condition is resolving. Increased central pain, decreased peripheral pain, and decreased neurologic signs are usually evidence that the compression of the spinal nerve root is decreased. A temporary increase in central pain may indicate a change in irritation to the nerve root.

Decreased pain together with increased neurologic signs indicate increased pressure to a nerve root, causing sensory deficits, motor weakness, or both. Document this outcome and contact the patient's physician. Decreased central pain coupled with increased peripheral pain indicate increased nerve root irritation.

Table 9–1 gives a general guide to modifying a traction treatment plan based on patient response to a previous traction session.

HOME USE

A variety of home traction devices are available for treatment of the cervical and lumbar regions. Patients may either rent or buy these devices. Devices generally differ in patient positioning requirements (i.e., supine, sitting, etc.) and

TABLE 9–1. General Guidelines for Treatment Modification

PATIENT SYMPTOMS	PATIENT SIGNS	ACTION
Improved	Improved	Keep the duration and pull unchanged. Be slow to increase if a joint is irritable. However, be sure to alter parameters if adequate improvement is not produced or maintained.
No change	No change	Either increase the duration, keeping the pull unchanged, or increase the pull, keeping the duration unchanged.
Improved	No change	Increase the duration, keeping the pull unchanged.
Improved	Worse	Keep the duration and pull unchanged.
Worse	Improved	Keep the duration and pull unchanged.
Worse	No change	Keep the duration unchanged and reduce the pull.
Worse	Worse	Either reduce the duration, keeping the pull unchanged, or reduce the pull, keeping the duration unchanged.

in the way that they provide a tractive force. Three commonly used means of delivering the traction force in home units are a pulley system using a water-filled bag, a pneumatic system where the patient pumps air into the system, or a rope and pulley system whereby the patient pulls the rope to create an auto-traction force. When choosing a home traction device, the clinician should consider patient positioning, patient safety, and whether the home traction device delivers sufficient therapeutic force.

REFERENCES

1. Saunders HD, Saunders R. Spine. *Evaluation, Treatment and Prevention of Musculoskeletal Disorders.* Vol 1. Chaska, Minn: The Saunders Group; 1995.
2. Colachis SC, Strohm BR. Cervical traction: relationship of traction time to varied tractive force with constant angle of pull. *Arch Phys Med Rehabil.* 1965;46:815–819.
3. Colachis SD, Strohm BR. Effect of duration of intermittent cervical traction on vertebral separation. *Arch Phys Med Rehabil.* 1966;47:353–359.
4. Colachis SC, Strohm BR. A study of tractive forces and angle of pull on vertebral interspaces in the cervical spine. *Arch Phys Med Rehabil.* 1965;46:820–830.
5. Colachis SC, Strohm BR. Effects of intermittent traction on separation of lumbar vertebrae. *Arch Phys Med Rehabil.* 1969;50:251–258.
6. Cyriax J. *Textbook of Orthopedic Medicine, Volume I: Diagnosis of Soft Tissue Lesions.* London: Ballière, Tindall; 1982.
7. Weatherell VF. Comparison of electromyographic activity in normal lumbar sacrospinalis musculature during static pelvic traction in two different positions. *J Orthop Sports Phys Ther.* 1987;8:381–390.
8. Hood CS, Hart DL, Smith HG, Davis H. Comparison of electromyographic activity in normal lumbar sacrospinalis musculature during continuous and intermittent pelvic traction. *J Orthop Sports Phys Ther.* 1981;2:137–141.
9. Onel D, Tuzlaci M, Sari H, Demir K. Computed tomographic investigation of the effect of traction on lumbar disc herniations. *Spine.* 1989;14:82–90.
10. Murphy MJ. Effects of cervical traction on muscle activity. *J Orthop Sports Phys Ther.* 1991;13:220–225.
11. Mathews JA. Dynamic discography: a study of lumbar traction. *Ann Phys Med.* 1968;9:275–279.
12. Gupta RC, Ramarao S. Epidurography in reduction of lumbar disc prolapse by traction. *Arch Phys Med Rehabil.* 1978;59:322–327.
13. Deets D, Hands KL, Hopps SS. Cervical traction: a comparison of sitting and supine positions. *Phys Ther.* 1977;57:255–261.
14. Harris PR. Cervical traction: review of literature and treatment guidelines. *Phys Ther.* 1977;57:910–914.
15. Finneson B. *Low Back Pain.* Philadelphia: J.B. Lippincott; 1973.
16. Saunders HD. Unilateral lumbar traction. *Phys Ther.* 1981;61:221–225.
17. Cyriax J. *Textbook of Orthopedic Medicine: Diagnosis of Soft Tissues Lesions.* 6th ed. Baltimore: Williams & Wilkins; 1975.
18. DeLacerda FG. Effect of angle of traction pull on upper trapezius muscle activity. *J Orthop Sports Phys Ther.* 1980;1:205–209.
19. Letchuman R, Deusinger R. Comparison of sacrospinalis myoelectric activity and pain levels in patients undergoing static and intermittent lumbar traction. *Spine.* 1993;18:1361–1365.
20. Cyriax J. *Treatment by Manipulation, Massage and Injection.* 10th ed. London: Ballière, Tindall; 1980.
21. Bard G, Jones M. Cineradiographic recording of traction of the cervical spine. *Arch Phys Med Rehabil.* 1964;45:403–406.
22. Goldie LF, Reichmann S. The biomechanical influence of traction on the cervical spine. *Scand J Rehabil Med.* 1977;9:31–34.

23. Judovich BD. Lumbar traction therapy and dissipated force factors. *Lancet.* 1954;74:411–414.
24. Matthews JA. The effects of spinal traction. *Physiotherapy.* 1972;58:64–66.
25. Beurskens AJHM, van der Heijden GJMG, de Vet HCW, et al. The efficacy of traction for lumbar back pain: a design of a randomized clinical trial. *J Manipulative Physiol Ther.* 1995;18(3):141–147.

ADDITIONAL READINGS

Andersson GBJ, Schultz AB, Nachemson AL. Intervertebral disc pressures during traction. *Scand J Rehabil Med.* 1983;9(suppl):88–91.

Beurskens AJHM, de Vet HCW, Koke AJA, et al. Efficacy of traction for non-specific low back pain: a randomized clinical trial. *Lancet.* 1995;346:1596–1600.

Jette DU, Falkel JE, Trombly C. Effect of intermittent, supine cervical traction on the myoelectric activity of the upper trapezius muscle in subjects with neck pain. *Phys Ther.* 1985;65:1173–1176.

Kisner C, Colby LA. The spine: traction procedures. In: Kisner C, Colby LA, eds. *Therapeutic Exercise: Foundations and Techniques.* 3rd ed. Philadelphia: F.A. Davis; 1995;575–592.

LeBan MM, Meerschaert JR. Quadriplegia following cervical traction in patients with occult epidural prostatic metastasis. *Arch Phys Med Rehabil.* 1975;56:455–458.

Manus-Garlinghouse N. Unilateral traction in conjunction with heat modalities, proper positioning, and exercises for a herniated nucleus pulposus: a case report. *Phys Ther.* 1985;65:1208–1210.

Pellecchia GL. Lumbar traction: a review of the literature. *J Orthop Sports Phys Ther.* 1994;20:262–267.

Petulla LR. Clinical observations with respect to progressive/regressive traction. *J Orthop Sports Phys Ther.* 1986;7:261–263.

Quain MB, Tecklin JS. Lumbar traction: its effect on respiration. *Phys Ther.* 1985;65:1343–1346.

Saunders HD. *Spinal Traction: A Continuing Education Module for Physical Therapists.* Lawrence: University of Kansas, Division of Continuing Education; 1979.

Saunders HD. Use of spinal traction in the treatment of neck and back conditions. *Clin Orthop.* 1983;179:31–38.

Stoner EK, Merry PH. Intra-abdominal pressure changes during lumbar traction. *Arch Phys Med Rehabil.* 1973;54:369.

Twomey LT. Sustained lumbar traction. An experimental study of long spine segments. *Spine.* 1985;10:146–149.

van der Heijden GJMG, Beurskens AJHM, Koes BW, et al. The efficacy of traction for back and neck pain: a systematic, blinded review of randomized clinical trial methods. *Phys Ther.* 1995;75(2):93–104.

Walker GL. Goodley polyaxial cervical traction: a new approach to a traditional treatment. *Phys Ther.* 1986;66:1255–1259.

Wong AM, Leong CP, Chen CM. The traction angle and cervical intervertebral separation. *Spine.* 1992;17:136–138.

Zylbergold RS, Piper MC. Cervical spine disorders. A comparison of three types of traction. *Spine.* 1985;10:867–871.

Electrical Stimulation

DESCRIPTION

Electrical stimulation is the use of an electrical current across the skin to excite nerve or muscle tissue. Stimulators are available as large multipurpose units as well as small portable units that may be worn on the belt. Some units are equipped with hand or foot switches that can trigger the onset or termination of the stimulation during functional activity. Electrical stimulation may be used to achieve many goals such as improved motor control, pain relief, and wound healing. This chapter deals with the use of electrical stimulation for goals involving motor activity.

PURPOSE AND EFFECTS

Electrical stimulation of individual muscles or muscle groups is a means of providing active exercise to muscles that the patient is unable to contract voluntarily. If the muscle is denervated, electrical stimulation may be able to maintain nutrition of the muscle through promoting blood flow, decreasing fibrotic changes in the muscle, and retarding denervation atrophy.[1-11] The research support for treating denervated muscle with electrical stimulation is not strong, however, and the technique is now used very little. If the muscle is innervated, neuromuscular electrical stimulation (NMES) can be used to:

1. Strengthen healthy muscle or muscle weakened by disuse atrophy by improving recruitment of motor units. Later, with sufficient muscle load, hypertrophy may occur.[12-16]
2. Facilitate improved motor recruitment during function (i.e., reeducation).[17,18] This application includes using NMES as an electrical orthosis

by providing appropriate muscle contraction at an appropriate place and time in a functional activity.[19,20]

3. Decrease spasticity through reciprocal innervation or a related mechanism.[21–24]
4. Maintain or improve mobility through repeated motion into the desired range.[25]
5. Improve endurance through improving the aerobic capacity of the muscle.[26–28]
6. Promote peripheral circulation through activating a muscle pump.[29,30]

INDICATIONS

1. Peripheral nerve injuries.
2. Tendon transplants.
3. Muscle inhibition due to joint pain and effusion.
4. Upper motor neuron lesions to reduce spasticity and facilitate active contraction.
5. Disuse atrophy to strengthen muscle.
6. Immobilization to assist venous and lymphatic drainage.
7. Orthopedic and neurologic conditions leading to limitation of range of motion.

CONTRAINDICATIONS

1. Where active motion is contraindicated (e.g., fusion, unfixated fracture, or recently sutured nerves or tendons).
2. Patients wearing demand-inhibited cardiac pacemakers. Chen maintains that the sensitivity of these pacemakers can be adjusted to allow patients wearing them to use electrical stimulation.[31]
3. Stimulation directly over superficial metal implants.
4. Active bleeding in the area to be treated.
5. Malignancies in the area to be treated.
6. Very disoriented patients.
7. First trimester of pregnancy.

PRECAUTIONS

1. Avoid treating over anesthetic skin whenever possible. If stimulation must be given over anesthetic skin, use lower intensities and observe the skin closely.
2. Avoid open wounds in the treatment area. Due to the loss of the highly resistant stratum corneum, current concentrates in the wound. Wounds are often treated with electrical current, but using electrical stimulation for motor goals involves amplitudes too high for safe use near denuded skin.
3. Avoid areas of extreme edema. The very conductive fluid prevents the current from reaching the target tissue.

4. Avoid areas in which heavy scarring or thick adipose tissue is present. These highly resistant tissues prevent the current from crossing the skin, and treatment may be painful to the patient.
5. Do not place electrodes over the laryngeal and pharyngeal muscles or near the carotid sinus.

INSTRUCTIONS

General Instructions for Using Electrical Stimulators

Prior to operating any electrical stimulator, be sure to have a thorough understanding of the equipment and how to prepare a patient for maximal safety and comfort.

1. For units that have a line cord, make sure that the cord is intact and that the plug is hospital grade.
2. Some units are battery operated. Be certain that batteries have a full charge and that the contacts are snug and free of corrosion.
3. Fuses are present in electrical equipment, both in the power circuit and the patient circuit. If the unit is on yet fails to operate, check to see if the fuses are intact.
4. Most stimulation currents are alternating currents or pulsed currents that change polarity with each half cycle. Consequently, polarity is rarely a question. When a unidirectional current is used, however, polarity of the treatment electrode must be selected. Polarity of the patient leads may be determined by their attachment to the terminals or by a polarity switch. Know the polarity of the lead wires. If the polarity of the wires is unknown and continuous direct current is used, drop both wires in a glass of water so that they are not touching each other. Apply current to the circuit and observe the tips of the leads. A large cluster of small bubbles of hydrogen gas forms at the cathode, and a few large bubbles of oxygen gas form at the anode.
5. All units have an amplitude control dial. Always be sure to set the amplitude control to zero before and after each procedure.
6. A meter to measure either current (milliamperes or microamperes) or voltage (microvolts) is present on some equipment. Know how to read the various scales.
7. Prepare the electrodes properly. Keep carbon- or silicon-impregnated rubber electrodes clean and cover them with a conductive gel before attaching them to the patient. Gel should be sufficient to cover the entire electrode evenly, without squeezing out around the perimeter when it is applied. Carbon- or silicon-impregnated rubber electrodes may be cut to shape if desired. Some pregelled adhesive electrodes require application of water, and others do not. Refer to the manufacturer's instructions for preparation of all electrodes.
8. The lead wires should be carefully maintained. Do not coil them tightly because such bending can break the conductor. Check the lead wires for breaks in the insulation, and make sure that they are secured to the electrodes carefully.

General Procedures

1. Instruct the patient about what to expect from treatment and what you expect of her.

2. The part of the patient to be stimulated should be clean and free of clothing and jewelry. Check the patient's skin integrity and sensation.

3. Reduce the patient's skin impedance at the stimulation site. Human skin may be either dry or oily, and either condition can increase the electrical impedance of the skin. Several possible methods reduce the impedance. If the skin is oily or the patient is wearing cosmetics, wash the skin with soap and water. Preheat dry skin to increase circulation and perspiration. Abrading dry skin slightly assists in removing scales. Clipping hair allows the current to reach the skin more easily. Suggest to patients that they refrain from the use of oils and lotions prior to treatment and from shaving the legs if treatment is to be delivered to the legs. Shaving can create discomfort from producing tiny openings in the skin that are highly conductive.

4. Select a stimulator and stimulus parameters appropriate for the condition of the muscle. The parameters to be adjusted include phase duration, current frequency, waveform, rise time, duty cycle, and ramp time. In general, a phase duration of 200 to 300 μsec for NMES is comfortable and efficient.[32–34] Select a waveform that provides an instantaneous rise time. A frequency of greater than 30 impulses per second is sufficient to produce a smooth, tetanic contraction in most muscles. Higher frequencies are fatiguing but more comfortable.[35] Select the frequency based on the goal of treatment and patient comfort. Specific suggestions of these and other parameters are listed below under headings related to various motor goals.

5. Position the patient comfortably and appropriately to allow access to the muscles to be stimulated. If possible, allow the patient to watch the procedures. Select a position that is most appropriate for the motor goal of treatment. It should allow the type of contraction that is necessary for the goal of treatment: that is, either isotonic or isometric. Specific suggestions are given below.

6. Describe the exact sensations to the patient before beginning treatment. Demonstrate the procedure on yourself if it will aid the patient's understanding.

7. Prepare the electrodes according to the general instructions and attach them to the lead wires and to the patient. Electrode contact should be smooth and firm but not compressive. Be certain that electrodes cannot come loose during treatment. Attach electrodes using body weight or with adhesive tape, tape patches, elastic wrap, or straps. If using body weight for electrode adhesion, be sure the patient does not lift his weight from the electrode, thereby breaking the circuit. Do not rely on self-adhesive electrodes to remain attached, especially if there is much patient movement.

8. There are two fundamental techniques of electrode placement. The unipolar technique of stimulation involves the use of one small, active electrode and one large, dispersive electrode. The same amount of current passes through each of them, but because of the smaller size of the active electrode, the current through it is much more dense, and the ef-

fects are stronger under the active electrode. The bipolar technique uses two equal-sized electrodes. With no difference in size, the density of the current is the same under both electrodes.

9. Electrode placement depends on the goal of treatment. In general, for NMES, place one or both of the electrodes over the motor point of the muscle(s) of interest. A motor point for a muscle is that point on the skin that overlies the band of motor end-plates. For a nerve, it is a point where the nerve is close to the skin. When the motor point is stimulated, as opposed to any other area of the muscle or nerve, a stronger response is observed. Although charts have been developed to assist in locating the motor points (see Appendix C), a thorough knowledge of the anatomy of muscles and their innervations is necessary to stimulate muscles most effectively. If the muscle has lost its physical connection with its nerve supply, the motor point no longer exists, and the muscle becomes equally excitable throughout.

10. To locate the motor point, place the electrode in the area of the motor point, and increase the current amplitude until a comfortable contraction is obtained. Note the amplitude and observe the quality of the contraction. If the contraction is not the desired response or if the patient complains of discomfort, turn the current down to zero, move the electrode to a nearby location, and return the current amplitude to the same level. Continue this procedure until you locate the site at which the contraction is the strongest at the same amplitude as the first contraction; this site is the motor point. Make sure that the correct muscle is responding. Because the skin impedance is lower at the motor point, patients frequently state that the stimulation feels better when the motor point is located.

11. Arrange the electrodes so that the current runs longitudinally through the muscle or muscle group.[36] To prevent short circuiting, electrodes should not touch each other or be closer to each other than the diameter of the smallest one.

12. Adjust the amplitude until a contraction of an appropriate size for the goal is observed. If the stimulator has a provision for a continuous flow of current (e.g., a constant current button), engage it during current adjustments. If not, adjust the amplitude only while the current is flowing and not when the current is off. Observe the contraction to be certain the correct muscle or group is responding in the desirable manner. If not, turn the amplitude to zero, move the electrodes, and repeat the procedure. When the proper contraction is obtained, adjust the amplitude to a level suitable for the goal of treatment.

13. Instruct the patient to try to work actively with the stimulation if this is consistent with the treatment goal. Manual exercises of the entire extremity may take place during the stimulation. Be certain that the electrodes are securely attached.

14. At the end of the treatment, turn the amplitude to zero before removing the electrodes from the skin. Remove the apparatus, and clean the patient.

15. Perform all indicated posttreatment evaluation procedures, including skin inspection.

16. Document the goal of treatment, electrical parameters used, dosage, and patient response.

Specific Goals of NMES

In the sections below, specific suggestions are made for various motor goals. To plan an intervention with NMES for a motor goal, many clinical decisions must be made about the patient, the characteristics of the stimuli, and the stimulation program. In some cases, the decisions are common to all motor goals for innervated muscle. For example, the optimal phase duration to recruit alpha motoneurons is 200 to 300 μsec. In the summaries below, only those patient, stimulus, or program parameters that are specific to the goal are included. Where a decision regarding the parameter is common to all NMES applications, or is guided by patient comfort rather than physiology, it is omitted.

Strengthening

Healthy muscle or muscle that is weakened from disuse can be strengthened with NMES by improving recruitment of motor units and later through hypertrophy.

- **Position.** Place the muscle at resting length or in a slightly lengthened range.[37,38] Avoid closed-packed positions.
- **Type of Contraction.** Greater tension is built in the muscle if contractions are isometric.[37] Due to the specificity of exercise, treat the patient at several points in the range of motion.[39]
- **Frequency.** Greater tension is built with higher frequencies, but they can be fatiguing. A frequency of 50 pulses per second (pps) provides as much tension production as higher frequencies.[35,40]
- **Amplitude.** Increase the amplitude until a strong, preferably maximal, contraction is obtained. Patient tolerance is the guide, and the stimulation should not be painful.
- **Duty Cycle.** A rest cycle that is five to six times as long as the hold cycle allows the muscle adequate time to recover between contractions and produce the same amount of tension on each subsequent contraction.[35,41] A hold time of 6 to 10 seconds builds optimal tension.[39]
- **Treatment Duration.** Eight to ten contractions in one treatment session are sufficient for strengthening.[42] Strength gains from motor unit recruitment probably peak in about 20 to 25 sessions.[43]
- **Treatment Frequency.** Provide treatments daily or every other day.[43]

Endurance

For optimal function, muscles often must contract repeatedly or for long periods. Enhancing this ability involves minimizing fatigue of the type II motor units and providing a simulated training stimulus whereby fatigue resistance can be built.

- **Frequency.** A minimal tetanizing frequency (less than 40 pps) minimizes fatigue and causes recruited motor units to behave like type I motor units.[28]
- **Duty Cycle.** The duty cycle should be related to the functional activity. To simulate a training effect, start with a nonfatiguing duty cycle such as 1:6 and progress toward longer "on" times or shorter "off" times.
- **Treatment Duration.** Start with a number of contractions that the patient can tolerate without excessive fatigue. To simulate a training effect,

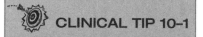

CLINICAL TIP 10–1

Decisions in Planning Interventions Using Neuromuscular Electrical Stimulation for Motor Goals

Patient
Principle of treatment
Type of contraction
Patient position

Stimulus
Waveform
Phase duration
Amplitude
Pulse frequency or rate
Modulation
Duty cycle
Ramp/fall times

Program
Treatment time
Number of treatment sessions
Progression

gradually add more contractions until the patient can sustain the activity for a time related to the functional activity.

- *Treatment Frequency.* Sessions may be one to three times per day. Increase the frequency as tolerated.

Facilitation or Reeducation

Facilitating muscle activity during function can be accomplished by assisting a voluntary contraction through enhanced sensory input or by ensuring that the contraction occurs at the appropriate time with the appropriate force, speed, range, and time to reach the peak force necessary for the functional activity of which it is a part.

- *Type of Contraction.* For most functional activities, movement is necessary to meet the goal, and so an isotonic contraction is appropriate. Be aware that when limb motion is produced, the return to the starting position is uncontrolled. Provide a means to protect the limb as it returns to the starting position.
- *Frequency.* Most facilitation applications require repeated activity, so select frequencies appropriate for improving endurance.
- *Amplitude.* Increase the amplitude to a level that approximates the size of contraction needed for the functional activity.
- *Technique.* Consider using a hand or foot switch to trigger stimulation at an appropriate time in the function. Each device with switch capability operates in a slightly different manner. Some trigger switches can be set to initiate stimulation either when activated or deactivated. Review the manufacturer's manual to become familiar with the switches.
- *Treatment Duration and Frequency.* Provide short, frequent treatment sessions (10 to 30 minutes two to three times a day), depending on the patient's mental and physical stamina.

Spasticity Reduction

On occasion, increased tone from an upper motor neuron lesion can impede functional movement. Tone can be decreased through NMES through a mechanism similar to reciprocal inhibition.[21]

- *Type of Contraction.* Generally, movement against increased tone is the goal, so an isotonic contraction of the nonspastic antagonistic muscle is needed. Provide a means to avoid overstretching the spastic muscle and to return to the starting position without facilitating the spastic muscles.[21]
- *Frequency.* Avoidance of fatigue is important, so provide a minimal tetanizing frequency.
- *Duty Cycle.* Provide a duty cycle that does not fatigue (e.g., 1:6).
- *Ramp Time.* Provide a gradual ramp and fall to avoid a quick stretch to the muscle, increasing the tone.
- *Treatment Duration.* Tone is usually decreased for about the same amount of time after treatment as the treatment duration (i.e., a 15-minute treatment produces about a 15-minute period of relaxation). Gear treatment duration to the desired period of decreased tone. Several weeks of treatment may be necessary before changes in tone are retained more permanently.
- *Treatment Frequency.* Perform the treatment prior to functional training activities as often as those activities are done.

Mobility

Range of motion can be increased with NMES by strengthening weak muscles. NMES can also be used once increased range has been achieved through other means by repeatedly moving the part through the new range. Using NMES allows an increase in the amount of treatment time without actual practitioner intervention.

- *Type of Contraction.* To maintain range of motion, movement into the desired range is necessary, so provide an isotonic contraction into the new range. An isometric contraction at the end of the new range may be added to help strengthen the muscles. Provide a means to limit the motion and to return to the starting position without facilitating the tight muscles.
- *Frequency.* Repeated contractions are necessary, so select a minimal tetanizing frequency.
- *Duty Cycle.* To avoid fatigue, start with a 1:6 duty cycle and progress the patient toward a 1:1 duty cycle. Provide 10 to 15 seconds of hold time.
- *Treatment Duration and Frequency.* Provide treatment for one-half to one hour daily or twice daily.

Peripheral Circulation

Peripheral circulation can be improved with NMES by intermittently activating the muscle pump around the circulatory network to increase metabolic demand.

- *Frequency.* A low tetanizing frequency (20 to 30 pps) has been shown to be most effective.[44]
- *Amplitude.* A contraction only 10% to 30% of maximal is sufficient.[29]
- *Duty Cycle.* Use a nonfatiguing duty cycle (e.g., 1:6).
- *Treatment Duration and Frequency.* Treatment may be given for 10 to 30 minutes as frequently as is comfortable for the patient.

Denervation

Stimulation of denervated muscle is done to retard atrophy.[1–11] To be successful, treatment must be initiated as soon after injury as possible, because atrophy that has already occurred cannot be reversed.[2,5,20] Electrical stimulation to denervated muscle has been shown to be effective in laboratory animals, but studies have not consistently demonstrated its effectiveness in humans.[5,10,45–48] The treatment can be uncomfortable, and patients may not adhere to the necessary parameters.

- *Patient Position.* If stretched, the muscle produces more tension.[6,49]
- *Type of Contraction.* Greater tension is built with an isometric contraction.[6,49]
- *Phase Duration.* For denervated muscles, a stimulus of long duration is necessary. If chronaxy for the muscle is known, then that duration is appropriate for stimulation. If chronaxy is not known, use a stimulus duration of greater than 100 msec. An alternating current (e.g., continuous square or sine wave) of 5 Hz can provide a phase duration of 100 msec and is preferable for the safety of the patient's skin. The use of continuous

direct current, interrupted manually using a switch on an interruptor handle, also provides such a stimulus.

- *Polarity.* If direct current is used, make the cathode the stimulating electrode.
- *Frequency.* More stimuli produce more tension, but frequency is governed by phase duration. A 100-msec phase duration can be delivered only 10 times per second, assuming no rest period between stimuli.
- *Rise Time.* Because denervated muscle does not accommodate, either a fast or slow rise time may be used.
- *Amplitude.* Increase the amplitude until a strong contraction is obtained.[2,6,7,49] Patient tolerance is the guide, and the stimulation should not be painful.
- *Length of Contraction.* The contraction should be held at least 2 seconds.[49] A longer period produces no further increase in tension in denervated muscle. Allow a rest period four to five times as long as the length of contraction.[50]
- *Treatment Duration.* Allow 10 to 25 contractions; the stronger the contraction, the fewer needed. With newly denervated muscles, smaller and fewer contractions may be necessary at first to avoid fatiguing the muscle.[3]
- *Treatment Frequency.* Electrical stimulation for denervated muscle should be done three times a day with at least 10 minutes of rest between sessions.[6]

RESPONSES TO TREATMENT AND TREATMENT MODIFICATION

The patient should experience tingling under one or both electrodes. The primary response of the patient to a program of electrical stimulation should be related to the goal of the intervention. Some evidence of achievement of the goal should be apparent within 1 to 2 weeks of treatment, depending on the goal. At the conclusion of treatment, the skin should show no changes in color or integrity. Occasionally, patients experience skin irritation from the adhesion of the electrodes or the conductive medium used. Treatment at these sites should be discontinued until the irritation is relieved; alternate electrode sites may be used. The practitioner may also investigate other methods of electrode adhesion and conductivity to prevent further irritation.

HOME USE

Most of the treatments described here can be carried out by the patient using a portable stimulator. Stimulators and electrode supplies are available through many vendors and may be rented or purchased. Instruct the patient concerning the settings, especially the amplitude adjustment, and be sure that she understands the goal. If the patient is to control progression of treatment, be sure that she understands the criteria for making a change, the stimulus or program characteristics to change, and the direction and magnitude of the change.

REFERENCES

1. Cole BG, Gardiner PF. Does electrical stimulation of denervated muscle, continued after reinnervation, influence recovery of contractile function? *Exp Neurol.* 1984;85:52–62.
2. Guttmann E, Guttmann L. The effect of galvanic exercise on denervated and re-innervated muscles in the rabbit. *J Neurol Neurosurg Psychiatry.* 1944;7:7–17.
3. Herbison GJ, Jaweed MM, Ditunno JF. Exercise therapies in peripheral neuropathies. *Arch Phys Med Rehabil.* 1983;64:201–205.
4. Herbison GJ, Teng C, Reyes T, Reyes O. Effect of electrical stimulation on denervated muscle of rat. *Arch Phys Med Rehabil.* 1971;52:516–522.
5. Jackson S. The role of galvanism in the treatment of denervated voluntary muscle in man. *Brain.* 1945;68:300–330.
6. Kosman AJ, Osborne SL, Ivy AC. The influence of duration and frequency of treatment in electrical stimulation of paralyzed muscle. *Arch Phys Med.* 1947;28:12–17.
7. Kosman AJ, Osborne SL, Ivy AC. The comparative effectiveness of various electrical currents in preventing muscle atrophy in the rat. *Arch Phys Med.* 1947;28:7–12.
8. Kosman AJ, Osborne SL, Ivy AC. Importance of current form and frequency in electrical stimulation of muscles. *Arch Phys Med.* 1948;29:559–562.
9. Kosman AJ, Wood EC, Osborne SL. Effect of electrical stimulation upon atrophy of partially denervated skeletal muscles of the rat. *Am J Physiol.* 1948;154:451–454.
10. Osborne SL. The retardation of atrophy in man by electrical stimulation of muscles. *Arch Phys Med.* 1951;32:523–528.
11. Pachter BR, Eberstein A, Goodgold J. Electrical stimulation effect on denervated skeletal myofibers in rats: a light and electron microscopic study. *Arch Phys Med Rehabil.* 1982;63:427–430.
12. Boutelle D, Smith B, Malone T. A strength study utilizing the Electro-Stim 180. *J Orthop Sports Phys Ther.* 1985;7:50–53.
13. Currier DP, Lehmann J, Lightfoot P. Electrical stimulation in exercise of the quadriceps femoris muscle. *Phys Ther.* 1979;59:1508–1511.
14. DeLitto A, Rose SJ, McKowen JM, et al. Electrical stimulation versus voluntary exercise in strengthening thigh musculature after anterior cruciate ligament surgery. *Phys Ther.* 1988;68:660–663.
15. Laughman RK, Youdas JW, Garrett TR, Chao EYS. Strength changes in the normal quadriceps femoris muscle as a result of electrical stimulation. *Phys Ther.* 1983;63:494–499.
16. Stefanovska A, Vodovnik L. Change in muscle force following electrical stimulation. *Scand J Rehabil Med.* 1985;17:141–146.
17. Baker LL, Parker K, Sanderson D. Neuromuscular electrical stimulation for the head-injured patient. *Phys Ther.* 1983;63:1967–1974.
18. Bowman BR, Baker LL, Waters RL. Positional feedback and electrical stimulation: an automated treatment for the hemiplegic wrist. *Arch Phys Med Rehabil.* 1979;60:497–502.
19. Liberson WF, Holmquest HJ, Scott D, Dow M. Functional electrotherapy: stimulation of the peroneal nerve synchronized with the swing phase of gait in hemiplegic patients. *Arch Phys Med Rehabil.* 1961;42:101–105.
20. Waters RL, McNeal D, Perry, J. Experimental correction of footdrop by electrical stimulation of the peroneal nerve. *J Bone Joint Surg.* 1975;57-A:1047–1054.
21. Alfieri V. Electrical treatment of spasticity. *Scand J Rehabil Med.* 1982;14:177–182.
22. Levine JG, Knott M, Kabat H. Relaxation of spasticity by electrical stimulation of the antagonist muscles. *Arch Phys Med.* 1952;33:668–673.
23. Shindo N, Jones R. Reciprocal patterned electrical stimulation of the lower limbs in severe spasticity. *Physiotherapy.* 1987;73:579–582.
24. Vodovnik L, Bowman BR, Winchester P. Effect of electrical stimulation on spasticity in hemiparetic patients. *Int Rehabil Med.* 1984;6:153–156.
25. Baker LL, Yeh C, Wilson D, Waters R. Electrical stimulation of the wrists and fingers for hemiplegic patients. *Phys Ther.* 1976;59:1495–1499.

26. Hudlicka O, Brown M, Cotter M, et al. The effect of long-term stimulation of fast muscles on their blood flow, metabolism and ability to withstand fatigue. *Pflügers Arch.* 1977;369:141–149.

27. Ikai M, Yabe K. Training effect of muscular endurance by means of voluntary and electrical stimulation. *Int Z Angewandte Physiol.* 1969;28:55–60.

28. Salmons S, Vrbova G. The influence of activity on some contractile characteristics of mammalian fast and slow muscles. *J Physiol.* 1969;201:535–549.

29. Currier DP, Petrilli CR, Threlkeld AJ. Effect of graded electrical stimulation on blood flow to healthy muscle. *Phys Ther.* 1986;66:937–943.

30. McMeeken J. Tissue temperature and blood flow: a research based overview of electrophysical modalities. *Aust J Physiother.* 1994;40(4):49–57.

31. Chen D, Mersamma P, Puliyodil PA, Monga TN. Cardiac pacemaker inhibition by transcutaneous electrical nerve stimulation. *Arch Phys Med Rehabil.* 1990;71:27–30.

32. Alon G, Allin J, Inbar GF. Optimization of pulse duration and pulse charge during transcutaneous electrical nerve stimulation. *Aust J Physiother.* 1983;29:195–201.

33. Gracanin F, Trnkoczy A. Optimal stimulus parameters for minimal pain in chronic stimulation of innervated muscle. *Arch Phys Med Rehabil.* 1975;56:243–249.

34. Vodovnik L, Long D, Regenos E, Lippay A. Pain response to different tetanizing currents. *Arch Phys Med Rehabil.* 1965;46:187–192.

35. Benton LA, Baker LL, Bowman BR, Waters RL. *Functional Electrical Stimulation: A Practical Clinical Guide.* Downey, Calif: Rancho Los Amigos Hospital; 1980.

36. Brooks ME, Smith EM, Currier DP. Effect of longitudinal versus transverse electrode placement on torque production by the quadriceps femoris muscle during neuromuscular electrical stimulation. *J Orthop Sports Phys Ther.* 1990;11:530–534.

37. Ganong WF. *Medical Physiology.* 8th ed. Los Altos, Calif: Lange Medical Publications; 1977.

38. Tachino K, Susaki T, Yamazaki T. Effect of electro-motor stimulation on the power production of a maximally stretched muscle. *Scand J Rehabil Med.* 1989;21:147–150.

39. Lindh M. Increase of muscle strength from isometric quadriceps exercises at different knee angles. *Scand J Rehabil Med.* 1979;11:33–36.

40. Rack PMH, Westbury DR. The effects of length and stimulus rate on tension in the isometric cat soleus muscle. *J Physiol.* 1969;204:443–460.

41. Baker LL, Cole K, Hart J, et al. Effects of duty cycle and frequency on muscle fatigue during isometric electrically stimulated quadriceps contractions [Abstract R-292]. *Phys Ther.* 1988;68:835.

42. Liu HI, Currier DP. Minimum number of repetitions for augmenting the tension developing capacity of muscle by electrical stimulation [Abstract R-073]. *Phys Ther.* 1985;65:683.

43. Kots J. Lecture notes from Canadian-Soviet Exchange Symposium on electrostimulation of skeletal muscles. Babkin I, Timtsenko N, trans. Montreal, Canada: Concordia University; 1977.

44. Mohr T, Akers TK, Wessman HC. Effects of high voltage stimulation on blood flow in the rat hind limb. *Phys Ther.* 1987;67:526–533.

45. Boonstra AM, Van Weerden TW, Eisma WH, et al. The effect of low-frequency electrical stimulation on denervation atrophy in man. *Scand J Rehabil Med.* 1987;19:127–134.

46. Doupe J, Barnes R, Kerr AS. The effect of electrical stimulation on the circulation and recovery of denervated muscle. *J Neurol Neurosurg Psychiatry.* 1943;6:136–140.

47. Mokrusch T, Neundörfer B. Electrotherapy of permanently denervated muscle—Long-term experience with a new method. *Eur J Phys Med Rehabil.* 1994;4:166–173.

48. Nix WA, Dahm M. The effect of isometric short-term electrical stimulation on denervated muscle. *Muscle Nerve.* 1987;10:136–143.

49. Wehrmacher WH, Thomson JD, Hines HM. Effects of electrical stimulation on denervated skeletal muscle. *Arch Phys Med.* 1945;26:261–266.

50. Cummings JP. Conservative management of peripheral nerve injuries utilizing selective electrical stimulation of denervated muscle with exponentially progressive current forms. *J Orthop Sports Phys Ther.* 1985;7:11–15.

ADDITIONAL READINGS

General

Binder-MacLeod SA, Guerin T. Preservation of force output through progressive reduction of stimulation frequency in human quadriceps femoris muscle. *Phys Ther.* 1990;70:619–625.

Binder-Macleod SA, McDermond LR. Changes in the force-frequency relationship of the human quadriceps femoris muscle following electrically and voluntarily induced fatigue. *Phys Ther.* 1992;72:95–104.

Delitto A, Strube MJ, Shulman AD, Minor SD. A study of discomfort with electrical stimulation. *Phys Ther.* 1992;72:410–424.

Greathouse DG, Nitz AJ, Matulionis DH, Currier DP. Effects of short-term electrical stimulation on the ultrastructure of rat skeletal muscles. *Phys Ther.* 1986;66:946–953.

Grimby G, Wigerstad-Lossing I. Comparison of high- and low-frequency muscle stimulators. *Arch Phys Med Rehabil.* 1989;70:835–838.

Howe T, Petterson T, Oldham J, et al. Making muscles grow as they are told. *Physiotherapy.* 1992;78:745–746.

Howson D. Peripheral neural excitability. *Phys Ther.* 1978;58:1467–1473.

Hultman E, Sjoholm H, Jaderholm-Ek I, Krynicki J. Evaluation of methods for electrical stimulation of human skeletal muscle in situ. *Pflügers Arch.* 1983;398:139–141.

Lieber RL. Skeletal muscle adaptability, III: muscle properties following chronic electrical stimulation. *Dev Med Child Neurol.* 1986;28:662–670.

Miller CR, Webers RL. The effects of ice massage on an individual's pain tolerance level to electrical stimulation. *J Orthop Sports Phys Ther.* 1990;12:105–109.

Munsat T, McNeal D, Waters RL. Effects of nerve stimulation on human muscle. *Arch Neurol.* 1976;33:608–617.

Sinacore DR, DeLitto A, King DS, Rose SJ. Type II fiber activation with electrical stimulation: a preliminary report. *Phys Ther.* 1990;70:416–422.

Stanish WD, Valiant GA, Bonen A, Belcastro AN. The effects of immobilization and of electrical stimulation on muscle glycogen and myofibrillar ATPase. *Can J Appl Sport Sci.* 1982;7:267–271.

Trimble MH, Enoka RM. Mechanisms underlying the training effects associated with neuromuscular electrical stimulation. *Phys Ther.* 1991;71:273–282.

Ward AR. Electrode coupling media for transcutaneous electrical nerve stimulation. *Aust J Physiother.* 1984;30:82–85.

Circulation and Edema

Clemente FR, Matulionis DH, Barron KW, Currier DP. Effect of motor neuromuscular electrical stimulation on microvascular perfusion of stimulated rat skeletal muscle. *Phys Ther.* 1991;71:397–406.

Cosgrove KA, Alon G, Bell SF, et al. The electrical effect of two commonly used clinical stimulators on traumatic edema in rats. *Phys Ther.* 1992;72:227–233.

Fahgri PD, Van Meerdervort HF, Glaser RM, Figoni SF. Electrical stimulation-induced contraction to reduce blood stasis during arthroplasty. *IEEE Trans Rehabil Eng.* 1997;5:62–69.

Hudlicka O, Brown MD, Egginton S, Dawson JM. Effect of long-term electrical stimulation on vascular supply and fatigue in chronically ischemic muscles. *J Appl Physiol.* 1994;77:1317–1324.

Indergand HJ, Morgan BJ. Effects of high-frequency transcutaneous electrical nerve stimulation on limb blood flow in healthy humans. *Phys Ther.* 1994;74:361–367.

Karnes JL, Mendel FC, Fish DR. Effects of low voltage pulsed current on edema formation in frog hind limbs following impact injury. *Phys Ther.* 1992;72:273–278.

Liu HI, Currier DP, Threlkeld AJ. Circulatory response of digital arteries associated with electrical stimulation of calf muscle in healthy subjects. *Phys Ther.* 1987;67:340–345.

Strengthening

Abdel-Moty E, Fishbain DA, Goldberg M, et al. Functional electrical stimulation treatment of postradiculopathy associated muscle weakness. *Arch Phys Med Rehabil.* 1994;75:680–686.

Alon G, McCombe SA, Koutsantonis S, et al. Comparison of the effects of electrical stimulation and exercise on abdominal musculature. *J Orthop Sports Phys Ther.* 1987;8:567–573.

Cox AM, Mendryk SW, Kramer JR, Hunka SM. Effect of electrode placement and rest interval between contractions on isometric knee extension torques induced by electrical stimulation at 100 Hz. *Physiother Can.* 1986;38:20–27.

Currier DP, Mann R. Muscular strength development by electrical stimulation in healthy individuals. *Phys Ther.* 1983;63:915–922.

Currier DP, Mann R. Pain complaint: comparison of electrical stimulation with conventional isometric exercise. *J Orthop Sports Phys Ther.* 1984;5:318–323.

DeDomenico G, Strauss GR. Maximum torque production in the quadriceps femoris muscle group using a variety of electrical stimulators. *Aust J Physiother.* 1986;32:51–56.

Delitto A, Rose SJ. Comparative comfort of three waveforms used in electrically eliciting quadriceps femoris muscle contractions. *Phys Ther.* 1986;66:1704–1707.

Delitto A, Rose SJ, McKowen JM, et al. Electrical stimulation versus voluntary exercise in strengthening thigh musculature after anterior cruciate ligament surgery. *Phys Ther.* 1988;68:660–663.

Delitto A, Snyder-Mackler L. Two theories of muscle strength augmentation using percutaneous electrical stimulation. *Phys Ther.* 1990;70:158–164.

Eriksson E, Haggmark T. Comparison of isometric muscle training and electrical stimulation supplementing isometric muscle training in the recovery after major knee ligament surgery. *Am J Sports Med.* 1979;7:169–171.

Godfrey CM, Jayawardena H, Quance TA, Walsh P. Comparison of electro-stimulation and isometric exercise in strengthening the quadriceps muscle. *Physiother Can.* 1979;31:265–267.

Goonan MR, Guerriero GP, Godfrey D, Weisberg J. The effects of electrical stimulation of normal abductor digiti quinti on strength. *J Orthop Sports Phys Ther.* 1985;6:343–346.

Halbach JW, Straus D. Comparison of electro-myo stimulation to isokinetic training in increasing power of the knee extensor mechanism. *J Orthop Sports Phys Ther.* 1980;2:20–24.

Hartsell HD. Electrical muscle stimulation and isometric exercise effects on selected quadriceps parameters. *J Orthop Sports Phys Ther.* 1986;8:203–209.

Johnson DH, Thurston P, Ashcroft PJ. The Russian technique of faradism in the treatment of chondromalacia patellae. *Physiother Can.* 1977;29:266–268.

Kramer JF. Effect of electrical stimulation current frequencies on isometric knee extension torque. *Phys Ther.* 1987;67:31–38.

Kramer JF, Lindsay D, Magee D, et al. Comparison of voluntary and electrical stimulation contraction torques. *J Orthop Sports Phys Ther.* 1984;5:324–331.

Kramer JF, Mendryk SW. Electrical stimulation as a strength improvement technique: a review. *J Orthop Sports Phys Ther.* 1982;4:91–98.

Kramer JF, Semple JE. Comparison of selected strengthening techniques for normal quadriceps. *Physiother Can.* 1983;35:300–304.

Kramer JF, Wessel J. Electrical activity and torque following electrical stimulation and voluntary contractions of quadriceps. *Physiother Can.* 1985;37:283–287.

Kubiak RJ, Whitman KM, Johnston RM. Changes in quadriceps femoris muscle strength using isometric exercise versus electrical stimulation. *J Orthop Sports Phys Ther.* 1987;8:537–541.

Lainey CG, Walmsley RP, Andrew GM. Effectiveness of exercise alone versus exercise and electrical stimulation in strengthening the quadriceps muscle. *Physiother Can.* 1983;35:5–11.

Lieber RL, Silva PD, Daniel DM. Equal effectiveness of electrical and volitional strength training for quadriceps femoris muscles after anterior cruciate ligament surgery. *J Orthop Res.* 1996;14:131–138.

McMiken D, Todd-Smith M, Thompson C. Strengthening of human quadriceps muscles by cutaneous electrical stimulation. *Scand J Rehabil Med.* 1983;15:25–28.

Milner-Brown HS, Miller RG. Muscle strengthening through electric stimulation combined with low-resistance weights in patients with neuromuscular disorders. *Arch Phys Med Rehabil.* 1988;69:20–24.

Nitz AJ, Dobner JJ. High intensity electrical stimulation effect on thigh musculature during immobilization for knee sprain: a case report. *Phys Ther.* 1987;67:219–222.

Nobbs LA, Rhodes EC. The effect of electrical stimulation and isokinetic exercise on muscular power of the quadriceps femoris. *J Orthop Sports Phys Ther.* 1986;8:260–268.

Owens J, Malone T. Treatment parameters of high frequency electrical stimulation as established on the Electrostim 180. *J Orthop Sports Phys Ther.* 1983;4:162–168.

Selkowitz D. Improvement in isometric strength of the quadriceps femoris muscle after training with electrical stimulation. *Phys Ther.* 1985;65:186–196.

Snyder-Mackler L, Delitto A, Bailey SL, Stralka S. Strength of the quadriceps femoris muscle and functional recovery after reconstruction of the anterior cruciate ligament. A prospective, randomized clinical trial of electrical stimulation. *J Bone Joint Surg.* 1995; 77-A: 1166–1173.

Snyder-Mackler L, Garrett M, Roberts M. A comparison of torque generating capabilities of three different electrical stimulating currents. *J Orthop Sports Phys Ther.* 1989;10:297–301.

Soo C, Currier DP, Threlkeld AJ. Augmenting voluntary torque of healthy muscle by optimization of electrical stimulation. *Phys Ther.* 1988;68:333–337.

Strauss GR, DeDomenico G. Torque production in human upper and lower limb muscles with voluntary and electrically stimulated contractions. *Aust J Physiother.* 1986;32:38–49.

Walmsley RP, Letts G, Vooys J. A comparison of torque generated by knee extension with a maximal voluntary muscle contraction vis-à-vis electrical stimulation. *J Orthop Sports Phys Ther.* 1984;6:10–17.

Wigerstad-Lossing I, Grimby G, Jonsson T, et al. Effects of electrical muscle stimulation combined with voluntary contractions after knee ligament surgery. *Med Sci Sports Exerc.* 1988;20:93–98.

Williams JGP, Street M. Sequential faradism in quadriceps rehabilitation. *Physiotherapy.* 1976;62:252–255.

Williams RA, Morrisey MC, Brewster CE. The effect of electrical stimulation on quadriceps strength and thigh circumference in meniscectomy patients. *J Orthop Sports Phys Ther.* 1986;8:143–146.

Wong RA. High voltage versus low voltage electrical stimulation: force of induced muscle contraction and perceived discomfort in healthy subjects. *Phys Ther.* 1986;66:1209–1214.

Endurance and Fatigue

Binder-MacLeod SA, Guerin T. Preservation of force output through progressive reduction of stimulation frequency in human quadriceps femoris muscle. *Phys Ther.* 1990;70:619–625.

Binder-Macleod SA, McDermond LR. Changes in the force-frequency relationship of the human quadriceps femoris muscle following electrically and voluntarily induced fatigue. *Phys Ther.* 1992;72:95–104.

Glaser RM, Petrofsky JS, Gruner JA, Green BA. Isometric strength and endurance of electrically stimulated leg muscles of quadriplegics. *Physiologist.* 1982; 25(31.11):253.

Grimby G, Nordwall A, Hulten B, Henriksson KG. Changes in histochemical profile of muscle after long-term electrical stimulation in patients with idiopathic scoliosis. *Scand J Rehabil Med.* 1985;17:191–196.

Isakov E, Mizrahi J, Graupe D, et al. Energy cost and physiological reactions to effort during activation of paraplegics by functional electrical stimulation. *Scand J Rehabil Med.* 1985;(supp 12):102–107.

McDonnell MK, Delitto A, Sinacore DR, Rose SJ. Electrically elicited fatigue test of the quadriceps femoris muscle: description and reliability. *Phys Ther.* 1987;67:941–945.

Packman-Braun R. Relationship between functional electrical stimulation duty cycle and fatigue in wrist extensor muscles of patients with hemiparesis. *Phys Ther.* 1988;68:52–56.

Parker MG, Berhold M, Brown R, et al. Fatigue response in human quadriceps femoris muscle during high frequency electrical stimulation. *J Orthop Sports Phys Ther.* 1986;7:145–153.

Peckham PH, Mortimer JT, Marsolais EB. Alteration in the force and fatigability of skeletal muscle in quadriplegic humans following exercise induced by chronic electrical stimulation. *Clin Orthop.* 1976;114:326–334.

Scoliosis Management

Axelgaard J. Transcutaneous electrical muscle stimulation for the treatment of progressive spinal curvature deformities. *Int Rehabil Med.* 1984;6:31–46.

Axelgaard J, Nordwall A, Brown JC. Correction of spinal curvatures by transcutaneous electrical muscle stimulation. *Spine.* 1983;8:463–481.

Bobechko WP, Herbert MA, Friedman HG. Electrospinal instrumentation for scoliosis: current status. *Orthop Clin North Am.* 1979;10:927–941.

Bradford DS, Tanguy A, Vanselow J. Surface electrical stimulation in the treatment of idiopathic scoliosis: preliminary results in 30 patients. *Spine.* 1983;8:757–764.

Brown JC, Axelgaard J, Howson DC. Multicenter trial of a noninvasive stimulation method for idiopathic scoliosis: a summary of early treatment results. *Spine.* 1984;9:382–387.

Bylund P, Aaro S, Gottfries B, Jansson E. Is lateral electric surface stimulation an effective treatment for scoliosis? *J Pediatr Orthop.* 1987;7:298–300.

Eckerson LF, Axelgaard J. Lateral electrical surface stimulation as an alternative to bracing in the treatment of idiopathic scoliosis: treatment protocol and patient acceptance. *Phys Ther.* 1984;64:483–490.

Kahanovitz N, Snow B, Pinter I. The comparative results of psychologic testing in scoliosis patients treated with electrical stimulation or bracing. *Spine.* 1984; 9:442–444.

Kahanovitz N, Weiser S. Lateral electrical surface stimulation (LESS) compliance in adolescent female scoliosis patients. *Spine.* 1986;11:753–755.

McCollough NC. Nonoperative treatment of idiopathic scoliosis using surface electrical stimulation. *Spine.* 1986;11:802–804.

O'Donnell CS, Bunnell WP, Betz RR, et al. Electrical stimulation in the treatment of idiopathic scoliosis. *Clin Orthop.* 1988;229:107–113.

Sensory-Motor Facilitation

Baker LL, Parker K. Neuromuscular electrical stimulation of the muscles surrounding the shoulder. *Phys Ther.* 1986;66:1930–1937.

Carmick J. Clinical use of neuromuscular electrical stimulation for children with cerebral palsy, Part 1: Lower extremity. *Phys Ther.* 1993;73:505–513.

Carmick J. Clinical use of neuromuscular electrical stimulation for children with cerebral palsy, Part 2: Upper extremity. *Phys Ther.* 1993;73:514–527.

Carmick J. Managing equinus in children with cerebral palsy: electrical stimulation to strengthen the triceps surae muscle. *Dev Med Child Neurol.* 1995;37:965–975.

Carmick J. Use of neuromuscular electrical stimulation and a dorsal wrist splint to improve the hand function of a child with spastic hemiparesis. *Phys Ther.* 1997;77:661–671.

Faghri PD, Rodgers MM, Glaser RM, et al. The effects of functional electrical stimulation on shoulder subluxation, arm function recovery, and shoulder pain in hemiplegic stroke patients. *Arch Phys Med Rehabil.* 1994;75:73–79.

Gotlin RS, Hershkowitz S, Juris PM, et al. Electrical stimulation effect on extensor lag and length of hospital stay after total knee arthroplasty. *Arch Phys Med Rehabil.* 1994;75:957–959.

Gracanin F. Functional electrical stimulation in external control of motor activity and movements of paralysed extremities. *Int Rehabil Med.* 1984;6:25–30.

Gruner JA, Glaser RM, Feinberg SD, et al. A system for evaluation and exercise-conditioning of paralyzed leg muscles. *J Rehabil Res Dev.* 1983;20:21–30.

Kraft GH, Fitts SS, Hammond MC. Techniques to improve function of the arm and hand in chronic hemiplegia. *Arch Phys Med Rehabil.* 1992;73:220–227.

Peckham PH, Mortimer JT. Restoration of hand function in the quadriplegic through electrical stimulation. In: Hambrecht FT, Reswick JB, eds. *Functional Electrical Stimulation: Applications in Neural Prostheses.* New York: Marcel Dekker; 1977:83–95.

Petrofsky JS, Glaser RM, Phillips CA, Gruner JA. The effects of electrically induced bicycle ergometer exercise on blood pressure and heart rate. *Physiologist.* 1982;25(31.12):253.

Petrofsky JS, Phillips CA. The use of functional electrical stimulation for rehabilitation of spinal cord injured patients. *Cent Nerv Syst Trauma.* 1984;1:57–73.

Teng EL, McNeal DR, Kralj A, Waters RL. Electrical stimulation and feedback training: effects on voluntary control of paretic muscles. *Arch Phys Med Rehabil.* 1976;57:228–232.

Vodovnik L, Bajd T, Krajl A, et al. Functional electrical stimulation for control of locomotor systems. *CRC Crit Rev Bioeng.* 1981;6(2):63–131.

Winchester P, Montgomery J, Bowman B, Hislop H. Effects of feedback stimulation training and cyclical electrical stimulation on knee extension in hemiparetic patients. *Phys Ther.* 1983;63:1096–1103.

Spasticity

Bajd T, Gregoric M, Vodovnik L, Benko H. Electrical stimulation in treating spasticity resulting from spinal cord injury. *Arch Phys Med Rehabil.* 1985;66:515–517.

Chan CWY. Some techniques for the relief of spasticity and their physiological basis. *Physiother Can.* 1986;38:85–89.

Dimitrijevic N, Sherwood A. Spasticity: medical and surgical treatment. *Neurology.* 1981; 30:19–27.

Fulbright JS. Electrical stimulation to reduce chronic toe-flexor hypertonicity: a case report. *Phys Ther.* 1984;64:523–525.

Vodovnik L, Bowman B, Hufford P. Effects of electrical stimulation on spinal spasticity. *Scand J Rehabil Med.* 1984;16:29–34.

Waters RL. The enigma of "carry-over." *Int Rehabil Med.* 1984;6:9–12.

Orthotic Substitution

Bajd T, Krajl A, Rajko T, et al. The use of a four-channel electrical stimulator as an ambulatory aid for paraplegic patients. *Phys Ther.* 1983;63:1116–1120.

Bajd T, Krajl A, Sega J, et al. Use of a two channel functional electrical stimulator to stand paraplegic patients. *Phys Ther.* 1981;61:526–527.

Carnstam B, Larrson L, Prevec TS. Improvement in gait following functional electrical stimulation. *Scand J Rehabil Med.* 1977;9:7–13.

Coburn B. Paraplegic ambulation: a systems point of view. *Int Rehabil Med.* 1984;6:19–24.

Dan B. One small step for paraplegics, a giant leap for bioengineering. *JAMA.* 1983;249:1113–1114.

Krajl A, Bajd T, Turk R, et al. Gait restoration in paraplegic patients: a feasibility demonstration using multichannel surface electrode FES. *J Rehabil Res Dev.* 1983;20:3–20.

Marsolais EB, Kobetic R. Functional walking in paralyzed patients by means of electrical stimulation. *Clin Orthop.* 1983;175:30–36.

Merletti R, Andina A, Galante M, Fulan I. Clinical experience of electric peroneal stimulators in 50 hemiparetic patients. *Scand J Rehabil Med.* 1979;11:111–121.

Merletti R, Zelaschi F, Latella D, et al. A control study of muscle force recovery in hemiparetic patients during treatment with functional electrical stimulation. *Scand J Rehabil Med.* 1978;10:147–154.

Tabeke K, Kukulka C, Narayan M, et al. Peroneal nerve stimulation in rehabilitation of the hemiplegic patient. *Arch Phys Med Rehabil.* 1975;56:237–240.

Denervation

Brevet A, Pinto E, Peacock J, Stockdale FE. Myosin synthesis increases by electrical stimulation of skeletal muscle cell cultures. *Science.* 1976;193:1152–1154.

Brown MC, Holland RL. A central role for denervated tissue in causing nerve sprouting. *Nature.* 1979;282:724–726.

Davis HL. Is electrostimulation beneficial to denervated muscles? A review of results from basic research. *Physiother Can.* 1983;35:306–312.

Hayes KW. Electrical stimulation and denervation: proposed program and equipment limitations. *Top Acute Care Trauma Rehabil.* 1988;3(1):27–37.

Herbison GJ, Jaweed MM, Ditunno JF. Acetylcholine sensitivity and fibrillation potentials in electrically stimulated crush-denervated rat skeletal muscle. *Arch Phys Med Rehabil.* 1983;64:217–220.

Herbison GJ, Teng C, Gordon EE. Electrical stimulation of reinnervating rat muscle. *Arch Phys Med Rehabil.* 1973;54:156–160.

Jaweed MM, Herbison GJ, Ditunno JF. Physical activity and inactivity influences on ^{14}C-Leucine incorporation in reinnervated rat gastrocnemius. *Arch Phys Med Rehabil.* 1982;63:28–31.

Marin EL, Vernick S, Friedmann LW. Carpal tunnel syndrome: median nerve stress test. *Arch Phys Med Rehabil.* 1983;64:206–208.

Merletti R, Repossi F, Richetta E, et al. Size and x-ray density of normal and denervated muscles of the human leg and forearm. *Int Rehabil Med.* 1986;8:82–89.

Schimrigk K, McLaughlin J, Gruniger W. The effect of electrical stimulation on the experimentally denervated rat muscle. *Scand J Rehabil Med.* 1977;9:55–60.

Smith EM, Steinberger WW. Effect of stimulus parameter variation on recruitment in denervated rabbit muscle. *Arch Phys Med Rehabil.* 1968;49:566–572.

Steinberger WW, Smith EM. Maintenance of denervated rabbit muscle with direct electrostimulation. *Arch Phys Med Rehabil.* 1968;49:573–577.

Younkin S, Brett R, Davey B, Younkin L. Substances moved by axonal transport and released by nerve stimulation have an innervation-like effect on muscles. *Science.* 1978;200:1292–1295.

Transcutaneous Electrical Nerve Stimulation

Russell A. Foley

Transcutaneous electrical nerve stimulation (TENS) is the generic name for a method of afferent nerve fiber stimulation designed to control pain. This approach of nerve activation, often called neuromodulation or neuroaugmentation, is now well recognized for management of pain syndromes found throughout the body.[1] Due to technologic advances, there is now a variety of TENS units designed for specific modes of application. The different modes are identified by their parameter ranges of amplitude, frequency, and pulse duration. Stimulators designed with these parameters are small, lightweight, battery powered, and portable, weighing only a few ounces. This modality is designed to relieve the subjective perceptual complaint of pain relating to dysfunction. This form of neuroaugmentation also modulates the objective reflexogenic and autonomic physiologic responses to nociception.[2–4]

Pain mechanisms can be described in clinical reasoning categories relating to (1) input to the central nervous system, (2) central processing including the spinal cord dorsal horn and the suprasegmental affective/emotional components, and (3) an output component.[5] Body tissues, regardless of location, have classic responses to injury. These include inflammation and repair in the target tissue. Inflammation activates the free nerve endings, producing pain fiber activation. Pain fiber activation is one example of an input component of nociception beginning with the local target tissue and terminating in the central nervous system.[6]

The second category is processing within the central nervous system. The dorsal horn is the first integration center of nociceptive input. Activation of second and third order neurons may eventually lead to pain perception in the cortex of the brain.[7,8]

The final component is the output response that includes the autonomic and somatic motor systems.[9,10] Sympathetic/autonomic responses may include skin temperature and vascular changes, and motor abnormalities, driven through the anterior horn cell, may include tremor, dystonia, or weakness.[11,12] These are the objective signs of the pathobiology of pain. The clinical reasoning categories address the complexity of the pain/dysfunction presentation, thereby promoting comprehensive treatment strategies.[13,14] Modulation of nociceptive input, pain processing and the autonomic/motor output responses to pain enhance treatment of the primary dysfunction.[4,15–19]

It is difficult to predict the effectiveness of TENS in various pain conditions, whether acute or chronic. Pain is an extremely complex, and many times frustrating, phenomenon.[20–24] However, the efficacy of TENS can be maximized by using an individualized approach to patient evaluation, appropriate parameter adjustment, optimal electrode placement, and patient education as it relates to the new pain sciences. Most importantly, TENS should be considered to be just one part of a comprehensive treatment program designed for the appropriate management of pain as it relates to dysfunction.[25–27]

A recent advance in TENS development focuses on outcome data.[28] This advance is a data input, storage, and retrieval system built into the TENS equipment. This recently released TENS unit attempts to validate several areas of interest, including stimulation parameters, general usage, and the overall effectiveness of TENS intervention. In addition, these data can be used to track patient adherence. The ability to analyze this type of information may increase the potential for successful treatment. Specific documentation features include:

- Percent of sessions with pain relief
- Number of sessions of use
- Average session length in hours and minutes
- Most frequent change in pain relief
- Most frequently used intensity range on Channel 1
- Most frequently used intensity range on Channel 2

The control panel for the data system is integrated within the front panel of the unit; this location allows for easy retrieval of information for patient medical record documentation.

Throughout the discussions that follow, the reader should remember that the mechanisms of action described are proposed based on available research. Much work remains to clarify the exact mechanisms. The broad descriptions provided reflect the most commonly accepted rationales and clinical approaches to TENS. Practitioners are encouraged to recognize that these guidelines do not limit parameter selection or electrode placement to the ranges or locations suggested. Creativity and a clinical reasoning/problem-solving approach are important for all modes of TENS if consistent success with this method is to be achieved. A summary of the characteristics of the modes of TENS is in Table 11–1.

INDICATIONS

Painful conditions of an acute or chronic nature.

CONTRAINDICATIONS

1. TENS is contraindicated in patients with demand-type cardiac pacemakers.[29]
2. The safety of TENS stimulation during pregnancy or delivery has not been determined.

TABLE 11–1. Summary of the Different Modes of TENS

MODE OF TENS	AMPLITUDE	PULSE DURATION	PULSE RATE	MECHANISM OF ACTION	ELECTRODE PLACEMENT	TECHNIQUE OF APPLICATION	ONSET OF RELIEF	WAVEFORM EXAMPLES
Conventional	Comfortable paresthesia; submotor response	Narrow (50–125 µsec)	High; 50–110 pps	Segmental gate; dorsal horn	Local area of pain/dysfunction; related spinal segment	30–60 min wearing time; reassess each hour	Fast immediate (5–10 min)	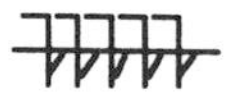
Low-frequency	Medium high; muscle fasciculation	Wide (200–500 µsec)	Low; 1–5 pps	β-endorphin	Segmentally related myotomes	40–60 min	Slow (20–40 min)	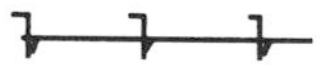
Burst	Medium high; muscle fasciculation	Wide (200–500 µsec)	High base rate (70–100 pps); Low burst rate (1–5 bps)	β-endorphin	Segmentally related myotomes	40–60 min	Slow (20–40 min)	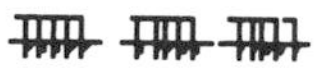
Modulation:								
• Conventional-like setup	Comfortable; low medium	50–125 µsec	High (85 pps)	Segmental gate; dorsal horn	Local area of pain/dysfunction; segmental spinal segment	30–60 min wearing time; reassess each hour	Fast immediate (5–10 min)	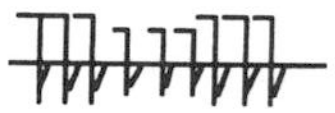
• Low-frequency–like setup	Combination adjustment: amplitude, pulse duration, rate with medium higher amplitudes with lower general rates; may include muscle fasciculation level amplitude			Descending inhibition; β-endorphin	Combination of local area of pain/dysfunction; segmentally related myotomes	Combination (20–60 min)	Medium slow (10–40 min)	
Preprogrammed regimens and strength–duration	Specific preprogrammed combinations of parameters			Any inclusion	Combination: local area of pain, segmental spinal, and distal sites	Combination (30–60 min)	Combination (fast [5–10 min] through medium-slow [10–40 min])	Bimodal 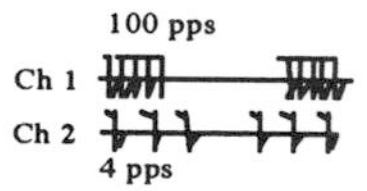100 pps Ch 1 Ch 2 4 pps Alternating ramped burst 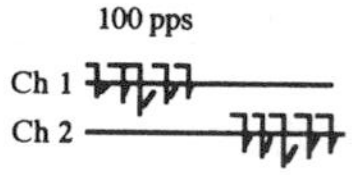100 pps Ch 1 Ch 2 Random modulation 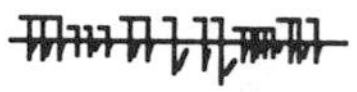 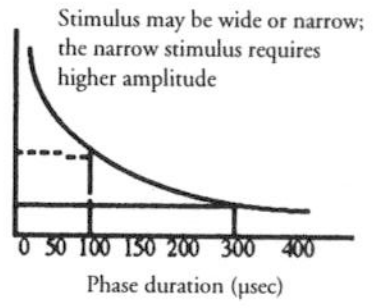Stimulus may be wide or narrow; the narrow stimulus requires higher amplitude 0 50 100 150 200 300 400 Phase duration (µsec)
Brief intense	High/strong paresthesia	Widest (250–400 µsec)	Highest (110–200 pps)	Axonal conduction block	Superficial peripheral nerves	15 min maximum	Instantaneous; fast (1–2 min)	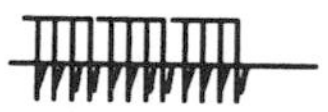
Hyperstimulation	High/noxious	250 µsec–10 msec	1–4 pps	Descending serotonin/enkephalin	Local acupuncture, trigger, or auricular point stimulation	30 seconds × 2 for each point; 10–20 points maximum	Fast (10 min); within 1–10 points	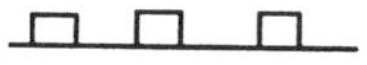

3. Stimulation sites over the carotid sinus, laryngeal or pharyngeal muscles, sensitive eye areas, or mucosal membranes should not be used.
4. TENS should not be used during operation of hazardous machinery.

PRECAUTIONS

1. TENS is designed for external use only.
2. TENS devices should be kept out of the reach of children.
3. Skin irritation may occur at the electrode placement sites.
4. TENS is not recommended for use by patients with known myocardial disease or arrhythmias without proper monitoring or safety precautions.

Conventional-Mode TENS

DESCRIPTION

Conventional-mode TENS is designed to provide a comfortable tingling sensation at a submotor level. The parameter ranges for this mode include pulse durations of 50 to 125 μsec, pulse rates of 50 to 110 pulses per second (pps), and a submotor amplitude that produces a paresthesia or tingling sensation.

PURPOSE AND EFFECTS

Conventional-mode TENS relieves pain through a proposed spinal cord gating mechanism.[30] Information regarding injury (nociception) is transmitted by free nerve endings to the central nervous system by peripheral nerves containing small diameter A-delta and C fibers.[31–34] These pain fibers enter the dorsal horn of the spinal cord and synapse with cells in various laminae, including lamina V. Information from the transmission (T) cells, located in lamina V, ascends the spinal cord to higher centers for autonomic responses and eventually perception as pain. The cells in the spinal cord that are excited by injury appear to be controlled by larger myelinated peripheral nerves carrying information about innocuous events. Input from mechanoreceptors is conveyed through these larger diameter A-beta and A-gamma fibers to the dorsal horn of the spinal cord.[35] These fibers synapse with cells in various laminae, including the substantia gelatinosa (SG), laminae II and III. Axon collaterals from the larger myelinated fibers excite the cells in the SG. Interneurons from the SG exert an inhibitory influence on the T cells of the pain fibers in lamina V.[30,36] These interneurons "close the gate" to pain transmission at the spinal cord level through a presynaptic or postsynaptic inhibitory event.[36] The interneurons that close the gate to pain transmission may involve a variety of neurochemical inhibitory processes using met-enkephalin or dynorphin through mu, delta, and kappa opioid receptors.[3,16,37–43] Conventional-mode TENS is an approach that activates the larger diameter peripheral nerve fibers to neuromodulate pain through a segmental spinal neurochemical gating mechanism.[44]

ADVANTAGES

1. Conventional-mode TENS is a neuromodulation approach that is usually perceived as comfortable by the patient.[36,45,46]
2. It has a relatively fast-acting mechanism of action; therefore, the effectiveness of selected parameters and electrode placement may be evaluated in a matter of minutes.
3. It may be used for both acute and chronic conditions, because the stimuli produce no motor responses.
4. The actual treatment time may be as long as 24 hours a day if appropriate for pain control. This length of stimulation is rarely used in a general patient population.

DISADVANTAGES

1. Based on a purely chemical (enkephalin) mechanism of action, the amount of time the patient is pain-free following each treatment session (carry-over) may be short, but this may be modified by other factors (e.g., breaking into the pain–muscle spasm/guarding cycle).[47,48]
2. Adaptation to the stimulus is common with conventional-mode TENS; therefore, increases in amplitude or pulse duration may be required to maintain the perceived paresthesia.

INSTRUCTIONS

1. Prepare the working area (i.e., equipment, tape, electrodes, etc).
2. Instruct the patient about what you are going to do, what to expect from treatment, and what you expect of him.
3. Preset each parameter for a specific value within the ranges for conventional-mode TENS; that is, a high rate and narrow pulse duration. The amplitude control should be in the "off" position.
4. Prepare the skin to ensure conductivity prior to electrode placement.
5. Plug the lead wires into the electrodes. Start with two electrodes. With most of their devices, manufacturers supply self-adhesive, disposable electrodes, which are conductive and convenient to use. Sterile disposable electrodes are also available for postoperative use. Prepare the electrodes as directed by the instructions found with the various electrodes.
6. Place the electrodes at the predetermined stimulation sites. There are numerous strategies for selecting appropriate electrode placement sites. It is important to perform a thorough evaluation of the patient to determine the relationship of the pain to the dysfunction or pathology. Once this relationship has been determined, electrode placement should follow at sites related to the dysfunction. These may include dermatomes, myotomes, paraspinal areas (recurrent meningeal nerve), motor points, myofascial trigger points, acupuncture points, or sclerotomes.

   Initially, the pair of electrodes may be placed surrounding the local area of pain if the location of the pain is at the area of dysfunction.

Electrodes should be positioned so that the paresthesia is felt within the area of the pain and dysfunction. Examples of electrode placements are presented in Figure 11–1.

If satisfactory pain reduction is not achieved with the initial placement, various combinations of distal or segmentally related sites may prove beneficial. An additional pair of electrodes may be used. Electrode placement may include the spinal segments that relate to the nociceptive afferent input to the spinal dorsal horn segment, with the electrodes placed at the apex of the paraspinal muscles. This location provides input to the posterior primary division of the spinal nerve, including the recurrent meningeal nerve. Stimulation at this site would drive dorsal horn inhibition at the segmental level of nociceptive input. This input may include somatic or visceral nociceptive afferent information.[14] Optimal stimulation sites may vary from treatment session to treatment session as well as from patient to patient.

7. Plug the lead wires into the TENS unit.
8. Turn the unit on and increase the amplitude to a comfortable setting. The patient should perceive a paresthesia below motor threshold. Based on the patient response, increase the amplitude until a small muscle contraction is observed. Then decrease the amplitude to a level just below the muscle contraction.
9. Generally, the effectiveness of the stimulation sites or selected parameter adjustments can be determined within 5 to 10 minutes. If the level of pain reduction is unsatisfactory, readjust the parameters within the available ranges, or change the stimulation sites over several treatment sessions. Reassessment and appropriate alterations ensure maximum efficacy with TENS. Once the most effective combination of electrode placement and stimulation parameters has been determined, treat the patient for 30 to 60 minutes.
10. At the end of the treatment time, turn the unit off and return all parameters to zero.
11. Remove the electrodes.
12. Perform all indicated posttreatment evaluation procedures, including skin inspection.
13. Document electrode placement, mode of TENS, stimulation parameters, duration of treatment, patient response, and follow-up instructions.

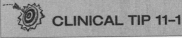

CLINICAL TIP 11–1

Options for Electrode Placement

Potential electrode placement sites include dermatomes, myotomes, paraspinal areas (recurrent meningeal nerve), motor points, myofascial trigger points, acupuncture points, or sclerotomes. Sometimes various electrode placement approaches may be combined into one placement or stimulation site. For example, the local area of pain may also include related dermatomes, myotomes, sclerotomes, myofascial trigger points, acupuncture points, or peripheral nerve trunks all directly related to the specific area of dysfunction or pathology. This multiple input approach using a single electrode placement is especially useful for the conventional, brief intense, modulation, and strength–duration modes of TENS.

DOSAGE

Intensity

The amplitude for conventional-mode TENS should be a comfortable sensation below motor threshold.

Duration

For most pain conditions, stimulation times range from 30 to 60 minutes. The general rule for wearing time is the minimal amount of stimulation time for the maximal amount of pain reduction. Some patients may require stimulation 24 hours a day (e.g., postoperative patients).

Problem	Electrode Placement	Rationale
Anterior right knee pain (could be of various origins, e.g., total knee replacement, prepatellar bursitis, patellofemoral dysfunction, patellar tendinitis)	Initial Placement - Superior-medial/Inferior-lateral (placement 1 in Figure 11-1A)	Encloses the local area of pain/dysfunction Structures at the anterior knee are innervated by L2,3,4; these dermatomes are included in this placement; peroneal nerve L4,5,S1,2 is also included. May include trigger points or acupuncture points
	Alternate Placement - if use dual channel, could add superior-lateral/inferior-medial (placement 2 in Figure 11-1A)	As above
	Alternate Placement - Paraspinal - either ipsilateral or crossed channel (placement 3 in Figure 11-1A)	Includes the posterior primary divisions and recurrent meningeal nerve for levels L2,3,4 This placement relates to the sensory-nociceptive information coming from the anterior knee to the segments of the spinal cord that innervate the knee (sclerotomes, dermatomes, myotomes, etc.)
	Alternate Placement - Combination of electrodes at the local area of pain and at the paraspinal segmental level	Combination of enclosing the local area of pain and stimulating the spinal segment
	Alternate Placement - Follow femoral (L2,3,4) or saphenous (L3,4) nerves from spinal segment to femoral triangle and then to knee	Can potentially combine spinal distribution and peripheral nerve distribution with local area of pain
Problem	**Electrode Placement**	**Rationale**
Low back pain with L4 nerve root pain on the left	Initial Placement - Ipsilaterally, contralaterally, or interferentially at or superior and inferior to the L4 spinal level (placement 1 in Figure 11-1B)	Includes local area of pain, posterior primary divisions L2,3,4,5,S1; and multisegmental recurrent meningeal nerves above and below the segment of involvement.
	Alternate Placement - Distal lower extremity with electrodes in the L4 dermatome (placement 2 in Figure 11-1B)	Will also include L4 myotome and can include the muscle motor point, acupuncture points or trigger points
	Alternate Placement - Along the sciatic nerve (placement 3 in Figure 11-1B)	Track peripheral nerve with L4 innervation; i.e., tibial (L4,5,S,1,2,3), peroneal (L4,5,S1,2)

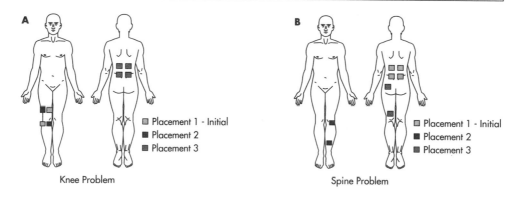

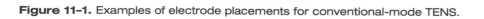

Figure 11–1. Examples of electrode placements for conventional-mode TENS.

Frequency

Generally, conventional-mode TENS is used daily, twice daily, or as often as needed. Adjust the frequency of use to maintain the patient in a pain-free state for as long as possible.

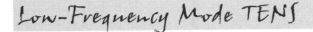

Low-Frequency Mode TENS

DESCRIPTION

Low-frequency mode TENS is used as another form of neuromodulation. This approach is also referred to as acupuncture-like TENS.[49,50] This mode of TENS is designed to recruit a variety of deep afferent nerves to produce central inhibitory effects through the endogenous opiates.[51] The parameter ranges for this mode include pulse durations of 200 to 500 μsec, pulse rates of 1 to 5 pps, and an amplitude strong enough to elicit a local muscle contraction in segmentally related myotomes. These stimulus parameters are opposite to those used for conventional-mode TENS, which uses a narrow duration, high frequency, and low amplitude.

PURPOSE AND EFFECTS

The analgesia produced by low-frequency mode TENS has been reversed by naloxone, a pure opiate antagonist.[50,52–56] Therefore, the mechanism of action appears to be related to a stimulation-evoked endogenous opiate. The stimuli introduced into the central nervous system initiate a sequence of events leading to the eventual release of β-endorphin.[42,55,57,58] It appears that low-frequency mode TENS stimulates the hypothalamus, which through releasing factors, stimulates the anterior and intermediate lobes of the pituitary gland. Found within the pituitary gland is a large prohormone precursor that breaks down to a 91–amino acid chain called β-lipotropin.[59–61] This 91–amino acid chain then fractions to a 31–amino chain called β-endorphin.[62,63] This endogenous morphine (β-endorphin) is released from the anterior and intermediate lobes of the pituitary and hypothalamus to bond with opiate receptors in the brain and spinal cord to produce an analgesic response.[8,37,64–66] There is also a corticotrophin sequence release from the β-lipotropin breakdown process, which in turn stimulates release of corticosteroid from the adrenal gland. This adrenal gland activation may produce an additional anti-inflammatory effect in the target tissue.

ADVANTAGES

1. The primary advantage of low-frequency mode TENS is the amount of time the patient is pain-free following each treatment session. The chemical half-life of β-endorphin is approximately 2 to 6 hours, which suggests a long-lasting analgesia following low-frequency TENS.[42,64]
2. Adaptation to the stimulus is slight; therefore, only minimal adjustment of amplitude and pulse duration is required to remain above motor threshold.[67]

DISADVANTAGES

1. A motor response is required to activate this form of chemical neuro-modulation. The muscle contraction may be perceived by patients as uncomfortable or annoying. Therefore, patients may not tolerate this mode of TENS.
2. In addition, the motor response may make this approach unsuitable for very acute pain conditions if the stimulation site is over the area of pain and dysfunction.
3. The motor response may limit the functional activities of the patient while undergoing stimulation.
4. To decrease the potential of any muscle soreness and fatigue produced by the repetitive contractions, the stimulation time is generally limited to 1 hour.
5. The onset of analgesia is delayed 20 to 30 minutes, allowing time for β-endorphin to be released into the system.

INSTRUCTIONS

1. Prepare the working area (i.e., equipment, tape, electrodes, etc).
2. Instruct the patient regarding the treatment and what you expect of her.
3. Preset the parameters for values appropriate to low-frequency mode TENS; that is, low rate and wide pulse duration. The amplitude control should be in the "off" position.
4. Prepare the skin to ensure conductivity prior to electrode placement.
5. Plug the lead wires into the electrodes. Start with two electrodes. With most of their devices, manufacturers supply self-adhesive, disposable electrodes, which are conductive and convenient to use. Sterile disposable electrodes are also available for postoperative use. Prepare the electrodes as directed by the instructions found with the various electrodes.
6. Place the electrodes at the predetermined stimulation sites. There are numerous strategies for selecting appropriate electrode placement sites. It is important to perform a thorough evaluation of the patient to determine the relationship of the pain to the dysfunction or pathology. Once this relationship has been determined, place the electrodes on sites that may include myotomes, paraspinal areas (recurrent meningeal nerve), motor points, myofascial trigger points, acupuncture points, peripheral nerve trunks, sclerotomes, or local areas of pain related to the dysfunction. A muscle contraction is necessary for this mode; therefore, the primary site is on the motor points of the muscles in the segmentally related myotome. Examples of electrode placement are presented in Figure 11–2.
7. Plug the lead wires into the unit.
8. Turn the unit on and increase the amplitude to elicit a strong, rhythmic muscle contraction. Intensities of this level may be perceived as uncomfortable by the patient. The induction time for opiate response, or analgesia, is approximately 20 to 30 minutes.

   Clinical practice has demonstrated that the use of conventional-mode TENS in conjunction with low-frequency mode TENS is benefi-

Problem	Electrode Placement	Rationale
Low back pain with L4 nerve root radiation into the right lower extremity	Initial Placement - Lower extremity over the anterolateral or anterior compartment (placement 1 in Figure 11-2)	Placement will include the L4 myotome the tibialis anterior, an L4 muscle. May also include trigger points, acupuncture points, the peripheral nerve distribution (peroneal). All allow input to L4 spinal segment.
	Alternate Placement - Second pair of electrodes as a mirror placement on the other leg (placement 2 in Figure 11-2)	Crossed inhibition at the contralateral dorsal horn related to the segment of input; i.e., L4
	Alternate Placement - Paraspinal - contralateral placement (placement 3 on Figure 11-2)	Includes the posterior primary divisions and recurrent meningeal nerve for levels L4 and any combination of levels above or below with recurrent meningeal nerves
	Alternate Placement - Placed over the femoral nerve; i.e., inguinal area	Has L2,3,4 components
	Alternate Placement - Placed over sciatic nerve; i.e., greater sciatic foramen	Has L4,5,S1,2,3 components (tibial and peroneal)
	Alternate Placement - Place anywhere in the L3,4,5 dermatomes (torso or extremities)	Allows extrasegmental input from segments above and below the L4 nerve root

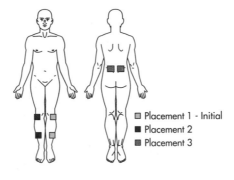

□ Placement 1 - Initial
■ Placement 2
■ Placement 3

Figure 11-2. Example of electrode placements for low-frequency mode TENS. Remember that muscle fasciculation in the segmentally related L4 myotome is necessary for low-frequency mode TENS.

cial. Initially, stimulate in the conventional mode for 10 to 20 minutes; then reset the parameters to low-frequency mode for the next 20 to 40 minutes. This approach will allow for initial comfort through a fast-acting gating mechanism, followed by a long-lasting analgesic mechanism.

9. At end of the treatment time, turn the unit off and return all parameters to zero.

10. Remove the electrodes.

11. Perform all indicated posttreatment evaluation procedures, including the skin inspection.

12. Document electrode placement, mode of TENS, stimulation parameters, duration of treatment, patient response, and follow-up instructions.

DOSAGE

Intensity

The amplitude must be high enough to elicit a strong, rhythmic muscle contraction.

Duration

The induction time for analgesia is approximately 20 to 30 minutes. Stimulation duration in the low-frequency mode should be limited to 1 hour to avoid muscle soreness and fatigue produced by the repetitive contractions.

Frequency

Stimulation is usually given once a day. The unit should then be turned off to evaluate the length of pain reduction. The frequency of treatment should be regulated to maintain the patient in a pain-free state for as long as possible.

Burst-Mode TENS

DESCRIPTION

Burst-mode TENS is quite similar to low-frequency mode TENS in its clinical response and mechanism of action. Burst-mode TENS uses a combination of high- and low-frequency pulses, as illustrated in Table 11–1. Each burst includes adjustable pulses at an internal carrier frequency of approximately 70 to 100 pps. Pulse durations for burst-mode TENS range from 200 to 500 μsec, burst rates are 1 to 5 bursts per second (bps), and the amplitude is set strong enough to produce local muscle contraction. This muscle contraction should occur in myotomes segmentally related to the area of dysfunction.[56]

PURPOSE AND EFFECTS

The analgesia produced by burst-mode TENS has been reversed by naloxone, a pure opiate antagonist. Therefore, the mechanism of action appears to be related to a stimulation-evoked endogenous opiate. The stimuli introduced into the central nervous system initiate a sequence of events leading to the eventual release of β-endorphin.[8] It appears that burst-mode TENS stimulates the hypothalamus, which through releasing factors, stimulates the anterior and intermediate lobes of the pituitary gland. Found within the pituitary gland is a large prohormone precursor that breaks down to a 91–amino acid chain called β-lipotropin. This 91–amino acid chain then fractions to a 31–amino acid chain called β-endorphin. This endogenous morphine (β-endorphin) is released from the anterior and intermediate lobes of the pituitary to bond with opiate receptors in the brain to produce an analgesic response.[42,58,68]

ADVANTAGES

1. The primary advantage of burst-mode TENS is the amount of time the patient is pain-free following each treatment session. The chemical half-life of β-endorphin is approximately 4 hours, which suggests a long-lasting analgesia following burst-mode TENS.[64,69-72]
2. The increased number of stimuli within the burst envelope appears to be more comfortable to the patient than the single stimulus associated with low-frequency mode TENS.
3. Adaptation to the stimulus is slight; therefore, only minimal adjustment of amplitude and pulse duration is required to remain above motor threshold.[67]

DISADVANTAGES

1. A motor response is required to activate this form of chemical neuromodulation. Some patients may consider the muscle contraction associated with burst-mode TENS to be annoying. However, patients generally feel that the muscle response with burst mode is more comfortable than the sensation perceived with single-pulse, low-frequency mode TENS.
2. In addition, the motor response may make this approach unsuitable for very acute pain conditions if the stimulation site is over the area of pain and dysfunction.
3. The onset of pain relief is delayed 20 to 30 minutes to allow time for β-endorphin to be released into the system.
4. To decrease the potential of muscle soreness and fatigue produced by the repetitive contractions, stimulation time is usually limited to 1 hour.

INSTRUCTIONS

1. Prepare the working area (i.e., equipment, tape, electrodes, etc).
2. Instruct the patient regarding the treatment and what you expect of him.
3. Set the parameters for values appropriate to burst-mode TENS; that is, low burst rate and long pulse duration. The amplitude control should be in the "off" position.
4. Continue the treatment as described for low-frequency mode TENS.

DOSAGE

Intensity

The amplitude must be high enough to elicit a strong, rhythmic muscle contraction.

Duration

The induction time for analgesia is approximately 20 to 30 minutes. Stimulation duration in the burst mode should be limited to 1 hour to avoid muscle soreness and fatigue produced by the repetitive contractions.

Frequency

Stimulation is usually given once a day. The unit should then be turned off to evaluate the length of pain reduction. The frequency of treatment should be regulated to maintain the patient in a pain-free state for as long as possible.

Brief Intense–Mode TENS

DESCRIPTION

Brief intense–mode TENS is designed to inhibit pain by using high ranges of frequency, pulse duration, and amplitude that are perceived as comfortable or tolerable by the patient.[42] Parameters are close to the limits of the available ranges including pulse duration at 250 µsec, frequency of 110 pps, and an amplitude to tolerance for maximum paresthesia. There may be slight nonrhythmic muscle contraction with this level of intensity.

PURPOSE AND EFFECTS

Brief intense–mode TENS is a very fast-acting form of neuromodulation. Electroanalgesia is almost immediate when the TENS unit is turned on. The mechanism of action appears to be a decrease in conduction along the A-delta and C fibers during stimulation, thus blocking the action potentials of nociception. This type of conduction block may produce an increase of potassium (K^+) in the periaxonal space, thereby inhibiting sodium (Na^+) transport and conductance.[7] Although there is a selective blockage of pain transmission, there appears to be a minimal loss of touch or pressure sensation.

ADVANTAGES

1. This form of stimulation is generally perceived as comfortable by the patient.
2. There is a very fast onset of analgesia, and therefore, evaluation of clinical effectiveness is almost immediate. This mode of TENS may be used for an extremely acute condition; the rationale is blockage of the pain-carrying nerve fibers.

DISADVANTAGES

1. Once the TENS unit is turned off, the return to normal sensation in the treatment area is quite rapid.
2. Because the length of treatment per session is 15 minutes, this mode may not be as effective for chronic pain problems compared to a longer treatment.
3. Electroanalgesia is greatest when electrodes are placed over major superficial peripheral nerves. Discomfort is more likely in an area with a signifi-

cant density of subcutaneous tissue overlying the nerves. Consequently, this mode is not as successful for back or neck pain.

4. Patients may perceive the higher intensities as annoying.

INDICATIONS

1. See those listed in the general discussion at the beginning of the chapter.
2. In addition, this mode of TENS may be used as an adjunct to deep friction massage (DFM) of a very localized area to manage discomfort of the massage technique (e.g., DFM for treatment of adhesions related to lateral epicondylitis).

CONTRAINDICATIONS AND PRECAUTIONS

1. See those listed in the general discussion at the beginning of the chapter.
2. In addition, by convention, treatment time must be limited to 15 minutes, because the mechanism of action is theoretically maintaining a conduction block of the nerve membrane.[16,48]

INSTRUCTIONS

1. Prepare the working area; (i.e., equipment, tape, electrodes, etc).
2. Instruct the patient about what you are going to do, what to expect from treatment, and what you expect of her.
3. Set the parameters for a specific value within the ranges for brief intense–mode TENS; that is, a high rate and long pulse duration. The amplitude control should be in the "off" position.
4. Prepare the skin to ensure conductivity prior to electrode placement.
5. Plug the lead wires into the electrodes. Start with two electrodes. With most of their devices, manufacturers supply self-adhesive, disposable electrodes, which are conductive and convenient to use. Sterile disposable electrodes are also available for postoperative use. Prepare the electrodes as directed by the instructions found with the various electrodes.
6. Place the electrodes at the predetermined stimulation sites. There are numerous strategies for selecting appropriate electrode placement sites. It is important to perform a thorough evaluation of the patient to determine the relationship of the pain to the dysfunction or pathology.

    Initially, if the pain is located in the area of the dysfunction, the pair of electrodes may be placed surrounding the local area of pain using major superficial peripheral nerves. Electrodes should be positioned so that the paresthesia is felt within the area of the pain and dysfunction. Generally, superficial peripheral nerves are the optimal stimulation site used with brief intense–mode TENS. An additional pair of electrodes may be used.
7. Plug the lead wires into the TENS unit.
8. Turn the unit on and increase the amplitude to a setting that produces a high level of paresthesia. The patient should perceive a paresthesia be-

low motor threshold. Based on the patient response, the amplitude may be increased until a muscle contraction is observed.

The effectiveness of the stimulation sites or selected parameters can usually be determined within several minutes. If the level of pain reduction is unsatisfactory, readjust the parameters within the available ranges, or change the stimulation sites over several treatment sessions. Reassessment and appropriate alterations ensure maximum efficacy with TENS.

9. For most pain conditions, stimulation time is 15 minutes. Brief intense–mode TENS is usually performed in a clinic setting rather than at home.
10. At the end of the treatment time, turn the unit off and return all parameters to zero.
11. Remove the electrodes.
12. Perform all indicated posttreatment evaluation procedures, including skin inspection.
13. Document electrode placement, mode of TENS, stimulation parameters, duration of treatment, patient response, and follow-up instructions.

DOSAGE

Intensity
The amplitude should produce a strong sensation below motor threshold. Based on the patient response, the amplitude may be increased until a muscle contraction is observed.

Duration
Stimulation time is usually 15 minutes.

Frequency
Brief intense–mode TENS may be repeated several times a day.

Modulation-Mode TENS

DESCRIPTION

Modulation-mode TENS provides a comfortable stimulus and cyclically modulates amplitude, pulse duration, and frequency. These parameters may be modulated in isolation or in combination (e.g., pulse duration and frequency). This type of paired modulation is known as multimodulation or combination modulation. The extent of the modulation combinations is dependent on the specific units of the various manufacturers. As many as 12 program options are available with some TENS machines. It has been proposed that these options provide varying outputs for customization to individual patient needs. This also allows for flexibility in parameter combinations to meet potential changing patient needs over time.

PURPOSE AND EFFECTS

Generally, modulation-mode TENS is designed to decrease nerve or perceptual adaptation to the stimulation that often occurs with constant, unchanging stimuli.[56,57,73] Modulation-mode TENS operates under the same principles and rationale as conventional-mode TENS. Refer to the conventional-mode TENS section.

ADVANTAGES

1. There is purportedly decreased nerve adaptation with modulation-mode TENS.
2. Modulation mode is preferred for some patients due to its perceived level of comfort.
3. It has a mechanism of action that is relatively fast acting; therefore, the effectiveness of a selected treatment setting may be evaluated in a matter of minutes.
4. It may be used for both acute and chronic conditions, because the stimuli produce no motor responses.
5. The actual stimulation time may be as long as 24 hours a day if appropriate for pain control. This length of stimulation is rarely used for a general patient population.

DISADVANTAGES

1. Based on a purely chemical (enkephalin) mechanism of action, the amount of time the patient is pain-free following each treatment session (carry-over) may be short. However, clinically, the carry-over may be fairly long based on other factors; for example, breaking into the pain–muscle spasm/guarding cycle.
2. Some patients may find the constantly changing stimulation annoying or actually uncomfortable.

INSTRUCTIONS

1. Prepare the working area (i.e., equipment, tape, electrodes, etc).
2. Instruct the patient about what you are going to do, what to expect from treatment, and what you expect of him.
3. Set each parameter for a specific value within the ranges for modulation-mode TENS; that is, a high rate and narrow pulse duration. The amplitude control should be in the "off" position. Place the mode selector switch into modulation or program position.
4. Prepare the skin to ensure conductivity prior to electrode placement.
5. Plug the lead wires into the electrodes. Start with two electrodes. With most of their devices, manufacturers supply self-adhesive, disposable electrodes, which are conductive and convenient to use. Sterile disposable electrodes are also available for postoperative use. Prepare the electrodes as directed by the instructions found with the various electrodes.

6. Place the electrodes at the predetermined stimulation sites. It is important to perform a thorough evaluation of the patient to determine the relationship of the pain to the dysfunction or pathology. Once this relationship has been determined, place electrodes at sites such as dermatomes, myotomes, paraspinal areas (recurrent meningeal nerve), motor points, myofascial trigger points, acupuncture points, peripheral nerve trunks, sclerotomes, or local areas of pain related to the dysfunction.

   Initially, if the pain is in the area of the dysfunction, the pair of electrodes may be placed surrounding the local area of pain. Electrodes should be positioned so that the paresthesia is felt within the area of the pain and dysfunction.

   If satisfactory pain reduction is not achieved with the initial placement, various combinations of distal and segmentally related sites may prove beneficial, or an additional pair of electrodes may be used. Optimal stimulation sites may vary from treatment session to treatment session as well as from patient to patient.

7. Plug the lead wires into the TENS unit.

8. Turn the unit on and increase the amplitude to a comfortable setting. The patient should perceive a paresthesia below motor threshold. Based on the patient response, the amplitude may be increased until a small muscle contraction is observed. Then decrease the amplitude to a level just below the muscle contraction.

   Generally, the effectiveness of the stimulation sites or selected parameter adjustments can be determined within 5 to 10 minutes. If the level of pain reduction is unsatisfactory, readjust the parameters within the available ranges, modify program modes, or change the stimulation sites over several treatment sessions. Reassessment and appropriate alterations ensure maximum efficacy with TENS.

9. For most pain conditions, stimulation times range from 30 to 60 minutes. A patient who responds with acceptable pain reduction may be instructed in a TENS home program.

10. At the end of the treatment time, turn the unit off and return all parameters to zero.

11. Remove the electrodes.

12. Perform all indicated posttreatment evaluation procedures, including skin inspection.

13. Document electrode placement, mode of TENS, stimulation parameters, duration of treatment, patient response, and follow-up instructions.

DOSAGE

Intensity

Modulation-mode stimulation should be comfortable and below motor threshold.

Duration

Stimulation times range from 30 to 60 minutes. The general rule for wearing time is the minimal amount of stimulation time for the maximal amount of pain reduction. Some patient populations may require stimulation 24 hours a day (e.g., postoperative patients).

Frequency

Generally, modulation-mode TENS is used daily, twice daily, or as often as needed. The frequency of treatments per day should be adjusted to maintain the patient in a pain-free state for as long as possible.

Strength–Duration Mode TENS

DESCRIPTION

Strength–duration (SD) mode TENS is another form of neuromodulation therapy. This mode of stimulation has a direct relationship to the SD curve of nerve excitability.[44] The microprocessor in the unit calculates an approximate SD curve based on the adjusted preset TENS parameter input. For example, the amplitude decreases 25% with a simultaneous increase in pulse duration of 32% over the preset control values. The percentage of value change becomes important in unit setup and instruction. Other units use an SD curve in all modes of stimulation, so that whenever the pulse duration control is adjusted, the intensity control range is changed to maintain a relatively constant strength of stimulation.[74]

PURPOSE AND EFFECTS

SD mode TENS is designed to track the normal SD curve, thereby providing maximum nerve firing in response to an external stimulus. Amplitude and pulse duration settings are individualized to the patient. In addition, this form of TENS should decrease adaptation that may occur with a constant stimulus.

ADVANTAGES

1. There is purportedly decreased nerve adaptation in response to the variable stimulus characteristics of SD mode.
2. SD mode TENS is preferred for some patients because they perceive it to be comfortable.
3. It has a relatively fast-acting mechanism of action; therefore, the effectiveness of selected treatment settings may be evaluated in a matter of minutes.
4. It may be used for both acute and chronic conditions, because the stimuli produce no motor responses.
5. The actual stimulation time may be as long as 24 hours a day if appropriate for pain control. This length of stimulation is rarely used for a general patient population.

DISADVANTAGE

Based on a purely chemical (enkephalin) mechanism of action, the amount of time the patient is pain-free following each treatment session (carry-over) may be short. However, clinically, the carry-over may be fairly long based on other factors; for example, breaking into the pain–muscle spasm/guarding cycle.

INSTRUCTIONS

1. Prepare the working area (i.e., equipment, tape, electrodes, etc).
2. Instruct the patient about what you are going to do, what to expect from treatment, and what you expect of her.
3. Set the parameters for a specific value within the ranges for SD–conventional-mode TENS; that is, a high rate and narrow pulse duration. The amplitude control should be in the "off" position. The function indicator switch should be set in the normal or conventional mode position.
4. Prepare the skin to ensure conductivity prior to electrode placement.
5. Plug the lead wires into the electrodes. Start with two electrodes. With most of their devices, manufacturers supply self-adhesive, disposable electrodes, which are conductive and convenient to use. Sterile disposable electrodes are also available for postoperative use. Prepare the electrodes as directed by the instructions found with the various electrodes.
6. Place the electrodes at the predetermined stimulation sites. It is important to perform a thorough evaluation of the patient to determine the relationship of the pain to the dysfunction or pathology. Once this relationship has been determined, place electrodes at sites such as dermatomes, myotomes, paraspinal areas (recurrent meningeal nerve), motor points, myofascial trigger points, acupuncture points, peripheral nerve trunks, sclerotomes, or local areas of pain related to the dysfunction.

   Initially, the pair of electrodes may be placed surrounding the local area of pain if the pain is in the area of dysfunction. Electrodes should be positioned so that the paresthesia is felt within the area of the pain and dysfunction.

   If satisfactory pain reduction is not achieved with the initial placement, various combinations of distal and segmentally related sites may prove beneficial, or an additional pair of electrodes may be used. Optimal stimulation sites may vary from treatment session to treatment session as well as from patient to patient.

7. Plug the lead wires into the TENS unit.
8. Follow the instructions for the SD mode as described in the instruction manual for the specific TENS unit. The information for SD mode adjustment varies from manufacturer to manufacturer.
9. The effectiveness of the stimulation sites or selected parameters can usually be determined within 5 to 10 minutes. If the level of pain reduction is unsatisfactory, readjust the parameters within the available ranges, or change the stimulation sites over several treatment sessions.

Reassessment and appropriate alterations ensure maximum efficacy with TENS.

For most pain conditions, stimulation times range from 30 to 60 minutes. A patient who responds with acceptable pain reduction may be instructed in a TENS home program.

10. At the end of the treatment time, turn the unit off and return all parameters to zero.
11. Remove the electrodes.
12. Perform all indicated posttreatment evaluation procedures, including skin inspection.
13. Document electrode placement, mode of TENS, stimulation parameters, duration of treatment, patient response, and follow-up instructions.

DOSAGE

Intensity

The amplitude in the SD mode should produce a comfortable sensation, below the level of muscle contraction.

Duration

The effectiveness of the stimulation can usually be determined within 5 to 10 minutes. Usually, stimulation times range from 30 to 60 minutes. The usual wearing time is the minimal amount of stimulation time for the maximal amount of pain reduction. Some patient populations may require stimulation 24 hours a day (e.g., postoperative patients).

Frequency

SD mode TENS is used daily, twice daily, or as often as needed. The frequency of daily use should be adjusted to maintain the patient in a pain-free state for as long as possible.

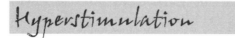

Hyperstimulation

DESCRIPTION

Hyperstimulation is a form of neuromodulation that uses noxious input to control pain.[36,74,75] In this approach, pain inhibits pain. The ranges of parameters for electrical hyperstimulation analgesia include pulse durations of 250 μsec to 10 msec, pulse rates of 1 to 4 pps, and an amplitude that produces the maximum tolerable level of noxious input. In addition to the specific parameters, noxious input is assured through the use of a small-diameter point-probe active electrode. The surface area of this electrode is small in comparison to the unit output, making the current density very high.

Hyperstimulation analgesia also may be produced by various techniques including dry needling, acupuncture, intense cold, intense heat, mechanical pressure, or chemical irritation of the skin.[30,36,72] Discussion here focuses on the use of handheld electrical probes for noninvasive (surface) stimulation. Frequently, units combine stimulation modes with skin resistance or "point locating" modes.[47,76–79] Points are usually identified through a meter reading or an audible signal. Once these points are identified, the unit is then switched into the stimulation mode for noxious input through electrical current.

PURPOSE AND EFFECTS

Hyperstimulation relieves pain through a proposed brainstem neurochemical mechanism that exerts descending inhibitory control at the spinal cord level. Noxious stimuli excite the smaller pain fibers leading to activation of the brainstem reticular formation. Information from the reticular formation then excites the midbrain periaqueductal gray (PAG),[74,80,81] an area with high opioid peptide concentration from the three opioid families including met-enkephalin, β-endorphin, and dynorphin.[58,82–85] The PAG activates the descending antinociceptive pathway from the raphe nucleus, which is high in serotonin concentration.[80,86–89] This descending pathway inhibits pain signals at the spinal cord level. This final segmental inhibition may be mediated by met-enkephalin–containing cells in laminae I, II, and V, dynorphin-containing cells in laminae I and V,[42,72,83,84,90,91] or direct serotonin postsynaptic effects in the dorsal horn laminae I, II, (III), and V. Thus, intense stimulation would activate small-diameter nerve fibers to block pain eventually; that is, pain inhibits pain.

ADVANTAGES

1. The analgesia produced by point stimulation frequently has a fast onset.
2. The effectiveness of this approach may be observed following stimulation of only a few points or in a matter of minutes.
3. The small active point electrode may be used in areas not conducive to placement of large electrodes adhered with tape or requiring a conductive medium (e.g., face, scalp, ear, or bony prominences).

DISADVANTAGES

The major disadvantage of this approach is the unpleasant noxious stimulation. Patients may not tolerate the intensities necessary to achieve an analgesic state.

INSTRUCTIONS

1. Prepare the working area (i.e., equipment, electrodes).
2. Instruct the patient regarding what to expect from the treatment and what you expect of him.
3. Technique for Point Location
   Initially points are "located" through an audible or metered mode.[92]
   a. Turn the unit on.
   b. Set the unit to audio or meter location mode.
   c. Calibrate the detection sensitivity of the machine. Apply the tip of the probe to the general area of the selected stimulation site.

    d. Have the patient hold the ground electrode.

    e. Adjust the machine to the skin sensitivity of the patient. The unit should now be adjusted for high or low (wet or dry) skin conductance to ensure a consistent baseline sensitivity setting.

    f. Move the probe slowly, with even pressure, over the approximate trigger point site. Continued readjustments of sensitivity may be required for accurate point location. Sensitivity should be increased or decreased to maintain the baseline threshold level. Areas of decreased electrical conductance should be adjusted to a more sensitive level.

    g. Continue moving the probe until the auditory signal or a maximum meter deflection identifies the point.

    h. Leave the probe on the point to stimulate it.

4. Stimulation Following Point Location

    a. Be sure that the output control is set at zero.

    b. Set the frequency in a range of 1 to 4 pps.

    c. Switch the unit to the stimulation mode.

    d. Increase the amplitude to maximum patient tolerance. Stimulate the point for 30 seconds. It may be necessary to readjust the amplitude during the stimulation to maintain a tolerable noxious input.

    e. Stimulate each point two times for 30 seconds each time. If the point appears to be hypersensitive, an additional 30 seconds of stimulation may be used. A hypersensitive point is an area that has significant conductance in the location mode and requires minimal amplitude in the treatment mode to produce a nociceptive response (see f (3) below).

    f. Three common responses may be observed with stimulation.

      (1) Latent pathologic points demonstrate a "breakthrough" phenomenon. These points initially tolerate the stimulus but become hypersensitive within 10 to 20 seconds. The stimulus intensity should be reduced when this breakthrough occurs, but maintenance of a noxious intensity should be continued.

      (2) Points that are not pathologic adapt to the stimuli, requiring continued amplitude increases to maintain noxious thresholds.

      (3) Optimal stimulation sites reach noxious threshold levels very quickly with a minimum amount of intensity. Minimal adaptation to the stimulation occurs at these hypersensitive points.

    g. Repeat the point location and stimulation procedure for each stimulation site.

    h. Stimulate a maximum of approximately 20 points per treatment. Treat the minimum number of points to achieve the maximum pain reduction.

    i. Start distally, or away from the acutely painful area, and gradually proceed toward the area of dysfunction as the condition resolves. Auricular points may be included if the practitioner prefers. An understanding of acupuncture point meridians enhances the success of the mode.

    j. Points that demonstrate high sensitivity to electrical stimulation are considered as optimal stimulation sites for subsequent treatment sessions.

5. Turn the unit off.

6. Perform all indicated posttreatment evaluations, including skin inspection.

7. Document electrode placement, mode of TENS, stimulation parameters, duration of treatment, patient response, and follow-up instructions.

DOSAGE

Intensity
The amplitude in hyperstimulation must produce a noxious sensation.

Duration
Each point is stimulated for 30 to 60 seconds.

Frequency
Initial treatments for painful conditions may be performed one to two times a day. As the latency of relief improves, treatment may be performed once daily or three to five times a week. The frequency of visits should be adjusted based on the individual patient's duration of pain relief.

RESPONSES TO TREATMENT AND TREATMENT MODIFICATION

The patient should experience tingling both under the electrodes and in an area related to the problems. For all modes of TENS, the primary response expected of the patient should be one of pain relief. The timing of pain relief has been discussed throughout this chapter and is summarized in Table 11–1. At the conclusion of treatment, the skin should show no changes in color or integrity. Occasionally, patients experience skin irritation from the adhesion of the electrodes or the conductive medium used. Treatment at these sites should be discontinued until the irritation is relieved; alternate electrode sites may be used. The practitioner may also investigate other methods of electrode adhesion and conductivity to prevent further irritation.

HOME USE

A patient who responds with acceptable pain reduction may be instructed in a TENS home program. Instruct the patient about stimulation parameters and electrode placement. Be sure to give additional instructions regarding skin care, how often to change the electrodes, whether to bathe with them on, and so on.

REFERENCES

1. Fields H. *Core Curriculum for Professional Education on Pain.* 2nd ed. Seattle: IASP Press; 1995.
2. Bonica JJ. Current concepts in post operative pain. *Hospital Practice.* New York: HP Publishing Co; 1978.
3. Dubner R, Hargreaves KM. The neurobiology of pain and its modulation. *Clin J Pain.* 1989;5(suppl 2):S1–S6.
4. Foley RA. TENS: back to basics. *Rehabil Manage.* 1989;2(4):41–46.

5. Gifford L, Butler D. The integration of pain sciences into clinical practice. *J Hand Ther.* April–June 1997:86–95.

6. Pritchett J. Substance P level in synovial fluid may predict pain relief after knee replacement. *J Bone Joint Surg.* 1997;1:114–116.

7. Group M, Stanton-Hicks M. Neuroanatomy and pathophysiology of pain related to spinal disorders. In: Modic MT, ed. *The Radiologic Clinics of North America: Imaging of the Spine.* 1991;29:665–673.

8. Hargreaves K, Dionne R. Evaluating endogenous mediators of pain and analgesia in clinical studies. In: Max MB, Portenoy RK, Laska EM, eds. *Advances in Pain Research and Therapy.* New York: Raven Press; 1991;18:579–598.

9. Campbell J. *Pain 1996—An Updated Review: Refresher Course Syllabus.* Seattle: IASP Press; 1996.

10. Janig W, Levine J, Michaelis M. Interactions of sympathetic and primary afferent neurons following nerve injury and tissue trauma. In: Kumaqawa T, Kurger L, Mizumura K, (eds). *Progress in Brain Research.* Amsterdam: Elsevier Science B.V.; 1996:113.

11. Janig W, Stanton-Hicks M. Reflex sympathetic dystrophy: a reappraisal. *Progress In Pain Research and Management.* Vol. 6. Seattle: IASP Press; 1996.

12. Jansen S, Turner J, Wiesenfeld-Hallin Z. Proceedings of the 8th World Congress on Pain. *Progress in Pain Research and Management.* Vol. 8. Seattle: IASP Press; 1997.

13. Jones M. Clinical reasoning in manual therapy. *Phys Ther.* 1992;72:875–884.

14. Foley, R. *Complex Regional Pain Syndromes: A Specialty Course Focusing on the Autonomic Nervous System.* Boulder, Colo: Neuro-Orthopedic Institute International, Longmans Pty Ltd, and Neuro-Orthopedic Press; 1998.

15. Augustinsson L, Bohlin P, Bundson P, et al. Pain relief during delivery by transcutaneous electrical nerve stimulation. *Pain.* 1977;4:59–65.

16. Benedetti C. Acute pain: a review of its effects and therapy with systemic opioids. In: Benedetti C, Chapman CR, Giron G, eds. *Advances in Pain Research and Therapy.* New York: Raven Press; 1990;14:367–424.

17. Zimmerman M. Peripheral and central nervous mechanisms of nociception, pain, and pain therapy: facts and hypothesis. In: Bonica JJ, Liebeskind J, Albe-Fessard DG, eds. *Advances in Pain Research and Therapy.* New York: Raven Press; 1979; 3:3–32.

18. Mayer R, Campbell J, Raga S. Peripheral neural mechanisms of nociception. In: Wall P, Melzack R, (eds). *Textbook of Pain.* 3rd ed. Edinburgh: Churchill Livingstone; 1994:13–44.

19. Gordan S, Dionne R, Brahim J, et al. Blockade of peripheral neuronal barrage reduces postoperative pain. *Pain.* 1997;70:209–215.

20. Fordyce WE. Environmental factors in the genesis of low back pain. In: Bonica JJ, Liebeskind J, Albe-Fessard DG, eds. *Advances in Pain Research and Therapy.* New York: Raven Press; 1979;3:659–666.

21. Inman V, Saunders J. Referred pain from skeletal structures. *J Nerv Ment Dis.* 1944; 99:660–667.

22. Wolf S, Mannheimer J, Foley R. *The relationship of TENS to reflex sympathetic dystrophy (RSD)-like symptoms.* Minneapolis, Minn: Medtronic Nortech Educational Series: Monograph; 1990.

23. Ramer M, Bisby M. Rapid sprouting of sympathetic axons in dorsal root ganglia of rats with a chronic constriction injury. *Pain.* 1997;70:237–244.

24. Raj P, ed. *Pain Medicine: A Comprehensive Review.* St. Louis: Mosby; 1996.

25. Cyriax J. *Textbook of Orthopedic Medicine.* 6th ed. Baltimore: Williams & Wilkins; 1975.

26. Gottlieb H, Strite L, Koller R, et al. Comprehensive rehabilitation of patients having chronic low back pain. *Arch Phys Med Rehabil.* 1977;58:101–108.

27. Kessler R, Hertling D. *Management of Common Musculoskeletal Disorders.* Philadelphia: Harper & Row; 1983.

28. EMPI. EPIX VT Quick Guide. St. Paul, MN: EMPI, Inc; 1998.

29. Chen D, Philip M, Philip P, Monga T. Cardiac pacemaker inhibition by transcutaneous electrical nerve stimulation. *Arch Phys Med Rehabil.* 1990;1:27–30.

30. Melzack R, Wall P. Pain mechanisms: a new theory. *Science.* 1965;150:971–979.

31. Angevine JB, Cotman CW. *Principles of Neuroanatomy.* New York: Oxford Press; 1981.

32. Bonica JJ. Applied anatomy relevant to pain. In: Bonica JJ, ed. *The Management of Pain.* 2nd ed. Philadelphia: Lea & Febiger; 1990;1:133–158.

33. Kerr FWL. Segmental circuitry and spinal cord nociceptive mechanisms. In: Bonica JJ, Albe-Fessard DG, eds. *Advances in Pain Research and Therapy.* New York: Raven Press; 1976;1:75–89.

34. Melzack R. The perception of pain. *Sci Am.* 1961;204:41–49.

35. Wyke B. Neurological mechanisms in the experience of pain. *Acupunct Electrother Res.* 1979;4:27–35.

36. Melzack R, Wall P. *The Challenge of Pain: Exciting Discoveries in the New Science of Pain Control.* New York: Basic Books; 1982.

37. Akil H, Bronstein D, Mansour A. Overview of the endogenous opioid systems: anatomical, biochemical and functional issues. In: Rodgers RJ, Cooper SJ, eds. *Endorphins, Opiates and Behavioral Processes.* New York: John Wiley & Sons; 1988:1–23.

38. Bonica JJ. Biochemistry and modulation of nociception and pain. In: Bonica JJ, ed. *The Management of Pain.* 2nd ed. Philadelphia: Lea & Febiger; 1990;1:95–121.

39. Frederickson RCA, Chipkin RE. Endogenous opioids and pain: status of human studies and new treatment concepts. In: Fields HL, Bessen JM, eds. *Progress in Brain Research.* Amsterdam: Elsevier Science; 1988;77:407–417.

40. Knapp J, Hawkins K, Lui G, et al. Multiple opioid receptors and novel ligands. In: Benedetti C, Chapman CR, Giron G, eds. *Advances in Pain Research and Therapy.* New York: Raven Press; 1990;14:45–85.

41. Kosterlitz HW, Paterson SJ. Opioid receptors and mechanisms of opioid analgesia. In: Benedetti C, Chapman CR, Giron G, eds. *Advances in Pain Research and Therapy.* New York: Raven Press; 1990;14:37–43.

42. Ramabadran K, Bansinath M. The role of endogenous opioid peptides in the regulation of pain. *Crit Rev Neurobiol.* 1990;6:13–32.

43. Tempel A. Localization and ontogeny of opioid peptides and receptors. In: Szekely J, Ramabadran K, eds. *Opioid Peptides: Biochemistry and Applied Physiology.* Boca Raton, Fla: CRC Press; 1982;IV:133–169.

44. Howson D. Peripheral neural excitability: implications for transcutaneous electrical nerve stimulation. *Phys Ther.* 1978;58:1467–1473.

45. Melzack R. Psychological concepts and methods for the control of pain. *Advances in Neurology.* New York: Raven Press; 1974;4:275–280.

46. Wall P. Modulation of pain by non-painful events. In: Bonica JJ, Albe-Fessard DG, eds. *Advances in Pain Research and Therapy.* New York: Raven Press; 1976;1:1–16.

47. Travell J, Rinzler SH. The myofascial genesis of pain. *Postgrad Med.* 1952;2:425–434.

48. Yaksh TL. Neurologic mechanisms of pain. In: Cousins MJ, Bridenbaugh PO, eds. *Neural Blockade in Clinical Anesthesia and Management of Pain.* Philadelphia: J.B. Lippincott; 1988:791–844.

49. Mannheimer C, Carlsson C. The analgesic effect of transcutaneous electrical nerve stimulation (TENS) in patients with rheumatoid arthritis: a comparative study of different pulse patterns. *Pain.* 1979;6:329–334.

50. Sjolund BH, Eriksson M, Loeser J. Transcutaneous and implanted electric stimulation of peripheral nerves. In: Bonica JJ, ed. *The Management of Pain.* Vol. 2. 2nd ed. Philadelphia: Lea & Febiger; 1990;1852–1861.

51. Andersson SA. Pain control by sensory stimulation. In: Bonica JJ, Liebeskind J, Albe-Fessard DG, eds. *Advances in Pain Research and Therapy.* New York: Raven Press; 1979;3:569–585.

52. Akil H, Mayer D, Liebeskind J. Antagonism of stimulation-produced analgesia by naloxone, a narcotic antagonist. *Science.* 1976;191:961–962.

53. Eriksson M, Sjolund B, Nielzen S. Long-term results of peripheral conditioning stimulation as an analgesia measure in chronic pain. *Pain.* 1979;6:335–347.

54. Mayer D, Price D, Rafii A. Antagonism of acupuncture analgesia in man by narcotic antagonist naloxone. *Brain Res.* 1977;121:368–372.

55. Sjolund BH, Eriksson MBE. Endorphins and analgesia produced by peripheral conditioning stimulation. In: Bonica JJ, Liebeskind J, Albe-Fessard DG, eds. *Advances in Pain Research and Therapy.* New York: Raven Press; 1979;3:587–592.

56. Woolf CF. Segmental afferent fibre-induced analgesia: transcutaneous electrical nerve stimulation (TENS) and vibration. In: Wall P, Melzack R, eds. *Textbook of Pain.* New York: Churchill Livingstone; 1989:884–896.

57. Mannheimer J, Lampe J. *Clinical Transcutaneous Electrical Nerve Stimulation.* Philadelphia: F. A. Davis; 1984.

58. Terenius L. Families of opioid peptides and classes of opioid receptors. In: Fields HL, Dubner R, Cervero R, eds. *Advances in Pain Research and Therapy.* New York: Raven Press; 1985;9:463–477.

59. Akil H, Richardson DE, Barcitas JD, Li C. Appearance of B-endorphin-like immunoreactivity in human ventricular cerebrospinal fluid upon analgesic electric stimulation. *Proc Nat Acad Sci.* 1978;75:5170–5172.

60. Bunney WE. Basic and clinical studies of endorphins. *Ann Intern Med.* 1979;91:239–250.

61. Goldstein A. Opioid peptides (endorphins) pituitary and brain. *Science.* 1976;193:1081–1086.

62. Snyder SH. Opiate receptors and internal opiates. *Sci Am.* 1977;236(3):44–56.

63. Terenius L. Endorphin in chronic pain. In: Bonica JJ, Liebeskind J, Albe-Fessard, DG, eds. *Advances in Pain Research and Therapy.* New York: Raven Press; 1979;3:459–471.

64. Bishop B. Pain: its physiology and rationale for management. Parts I, II, III. *Phys Ther.* 1980; 60(1):13–37.

65. Fields HL. Neural mechanisms of opiate analgesia. In: Fields H, Dubner R, Cervero F, eds. *Advances in Pain Research and Therapy.* New York: Raven Press; 1985;9:479–486.

66. Mao L, Han J. Peptide antagonist of delta-opioid receptor attenuates inhibition of spinal nociceptive reflex induced by stimulation of arcuate nucleus of the hypothalamus. *Peptides.* 1990;11:1045–1047.

67. Spielholz N, Nolan M. Conventional TENS and the phenomena of accommodation, adaptation, habituation and electrode polarization. *J Clin Electrophysiol.* 1995;1:16–19.

68. Millan MJ. Multiple opioid systems and pain. *Pain.* 1986;27:303–347.

69. Liebeskind J, Mayer D, Akil H. Central mechanisms of pain inhibition: studies of analgesia from focal brain stimulation. *Advances in Neurology.* New York: Raven Press; 1974;4:261–268.

70. Mayer DJ. Endogenous analgesic systems: neural and behavioral mechanisms. In: Bonica JJ, Liebeskind J, Albe-Fessard DG, eds. *Advances in Pain Research and Therapy.* New York: Raven Press; 1979;3:385–410.

71. Snyder SH. The opiate receptor and morphine-like peptides in the brain. *Am J Psychiatry.* 1978;135:645–652.

72. Yaksh TL. Central nervous system sites mediating opiate analgesia. In: Bonica JJ, Liebeskind J, Albe-Fessard DG, eds. *Advances in Pain Research and Therapy.* New York: Raven Press; 1979;3:411–426.

73. Melzack R. Folk medicine and the sensory modulation of pain. In: Wall P, Melzack R, eds. *Textbook of Pain.* New York: Churchill Livingstone; 1989;897–905.

74. Fields HL, Basbaum AI. Anatomy and physiology of a descending pain control system. In: Bonica JJ, Liebeskind J, Albe-Fessard DG, eds. *Advances in Pain Research and Therapy.* New York: Raven Press; 1979;3:427–440.

75. Takeshige C, Luo CP, Kamada Y, et al. Relationship between midbrain neurons (periaqueductal central gray and midbrain reticular formation) and acupuncture analgesia, animal hypnosis. In: Bonica JJ, Liebeskind J, Albe-Fessard DG, eds. *Advances in Pain Research and Therapy.* New York: Raven Press; 1979;3:615–621.

76. Melzack R. Myofascial trigger points: relations to acupuncture and mechanisms of pain. *Arch Phys Med Rehabil.* 1981;62:114–117.

77. Melzack R. Prolonged relief of pain by brief, intense transcutaneous somatic stimulation. *Pain.* 1975;1:357–373.

78. Vandershot L. Trigger points vs. acupuncture points. *Am J Acupunct.* 1976;4:233–238.

79. Melzack R, Stillwell DM, Fox EJ. Trigger points and acupuncture points for pain: correlation and implications. *Pain.* 1977;33:3–23.

80. Cheng R, Pomeranz B. Electroacupuncture analgesia could be mediated by at least two pain-relieving mechanisms; endorphin and non-endorphin systems. *Life Sci.* 1979; 25:1957–1962.

81. Hosobuchi Y, Rossier J, Bloom F, Guillemin R. Periaqueductal gray stimulation for pain suppression in humans. In: Bonica JJ, Liebeskind J, Albe-Fessard DG, eds. *Advances in Pain Research and Therapy.* New York: Raven Press; 1979;3:515–523.

82. Han J. Central neurotransmitters and acupuncture analgesia. In: Pomeranz B, Stux G, eds. *Scientific Basis of Acupuncture.* Berlin: Springer-Verlag; 1991:7–33.

83. Herz A, Millan MJ. Endogenous opioid peptides in the descending control of nociceptive responses of spinal dorsal horn neurons. In: Fields HL, Besson JM, eds. *Progress in Brain Research.* Amsterdam: Elsevier Science; 1988;77:263–273.

84. Hope PJ, Fleetwood-Walker SM, Mitchell R. Distinct antinociceptive actions mediated by different opioid receptors in the region of lamina I and laminae III–V of the dorsal horn of the rat. *Br J Pharm.* 1990;101:477–483.

85. Mayer D, Hayes R. Stimulation-produced analgesia: development of tolerance and cross-tolerance to morphine. *Science.* 1975;188:941–943.

86. Akil H, Mayer D. Antagonism of stimulation-produced analgesia by p-CPA, a serotonin synthesis inhibitor. *Brain Res.* 1973;44:692–697.

87. Akil H, Liebeskind J. Monoaminergic mechanisms of stimulation-produced analgesia. *Brain Res.* 1975;94:279–296.

88. Fields HL, Basbaum AI. Brainstem control of spinal pain-transmission neurons. *Annu Rev Physiol.* 1978;40:217–248.

89. Mayer D, Liebeskind J. Pain reduction by focal electrical stimulation of the brain: an anatomical and behavioral analysis. *Brain Res.* 1974;68:73–93.

90. Goldstein A, Tachibana S, Lowney L, et al. Dynorphin (1-13), an extraordinarily potent opioid peptide. *Proc Nat Acad Sci.* 1979;76:6666–6670.

91. Kajander K, Yoshinori S, Iadarola M, Bennett G. Dynorphin increases in the dorsal spinal cord in rats with a painful peripheral neuropathy. *Peptides.* 1990;11:719–728.

92. Castel JC. *Management of Pain with Noninvasive Acupuncture Therapy.* Lake Bluff, Ill: Neuromed; 1979.

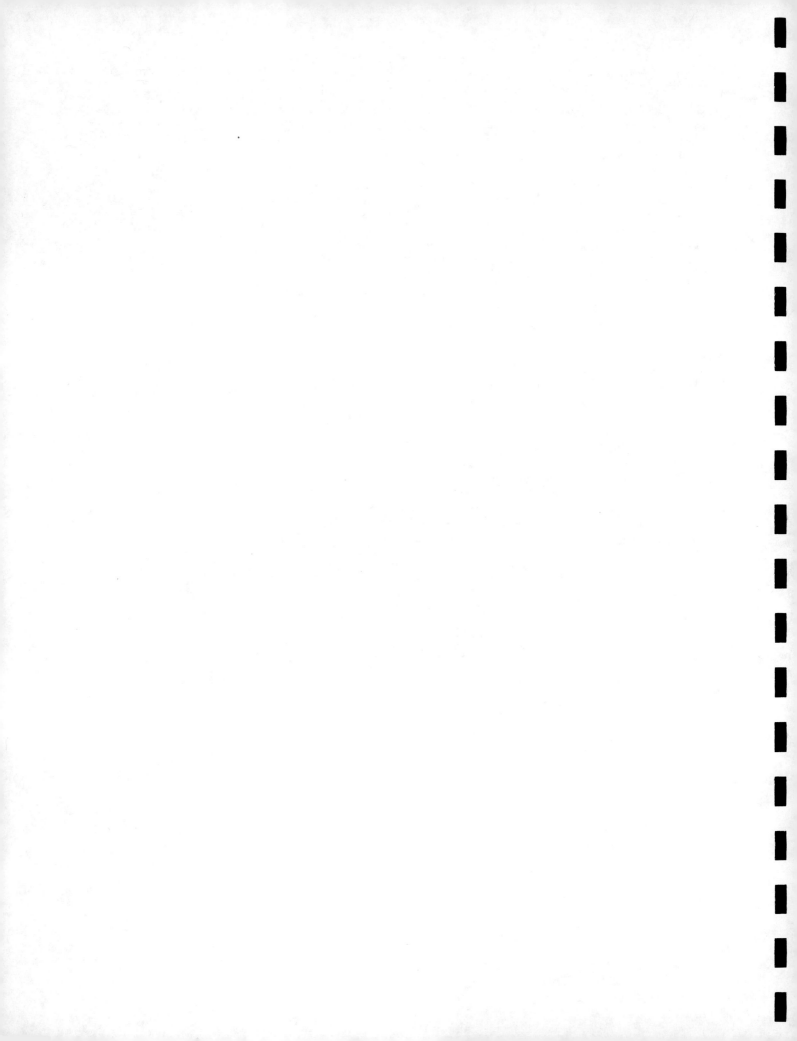

Interferential Stimulation

DESCRIPTION

Interferential stimulation is a treatment technique that uses medium-frequency currents. Theoretically, higher frequencies face less skin impedance and consequently are more comfortable. The type of treatment involves crossing the pathways of two unmodulated sine waves of different frequencies. Because of the different frequencies, the wave trains will arrive in phase at some points in time (constructive interference) and out of phase at other moments (destructive interference) where the paths cross. When the wave trains are superimposed, the combined amplitude is the sum of the individual wave train amplitudes; the amplitude is large when waves are in phase. In theory, the amplitude is zero when the waves are perfectly out of phase, but the waves may in actuality never be perfectly out of phase, so the destructive interference is not complete.[1] The result of the interference is an amplitude modulated sine wave. The frequency of the resultant wave train is between the frequencies of the incoming wave trains; if the amplitudes are equal, the resultant frequency is the average of the two incoming frequencies.[2] The modulation or beat frequency in beats per second is the difference between the frequencies of the incoming waves (Figure 12–1). For example, if the first circuit uses a 4000-Hz current, and the second circuit uses a 4100-Hz current, the resultant beat frequency is 100 beats per second.

Interferential current generators commonly use carrier frequencies of 2000 to 5000 Hz, with beat frequencies ranging from 0 to 1000 beats per second. When using a 4000-Hz frequency, the phase duration is 125 μsec, which is appropriate for both sensory and motor nerve stimulation, although its short phase duration makes it better for sensory nerve stimulation. When a longer phase duration is desirable for motor stimulation, the 2000-Hz carrier frequency may be more effective because of its 250-μsec width.

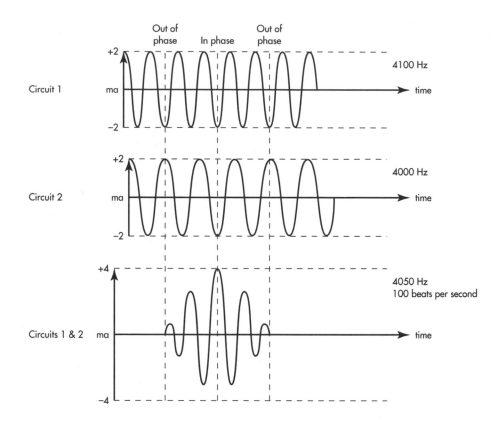

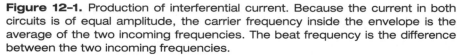

Figure 12-1. Production of interferential current. Because the current in both circuits is of equal amplitude, the carrier frequency inside the envelope is the average of the two incoming frequencies. The beat frequency is the difference between the two incoming frequencies.

The frequency of the second circuit can be fixed at a single frequency or allowed to vary automatically through a range of frequencies. This frequency modulation is often called frequency sweep or swing. This variable frequency purportedly prevents adaptation. There is some indication that certain swing patterns may be more effective than others,[3] but the efficacy of such variation is not well studied.

In a homogeneous medium, the resultant current is thought to be produced in a cloverleaf-shaped pattern with the maximal stimulation being produced on a diagonal between the circuit paths (Figure 12–2). The angle is 45 degrees if the amplitudes of the two circuits are equal. If the amplitudes are not equal, the resultant diagonal shifts to another angle.

Some equipment allows automatic increase and decrease of the amplitude of the second circuit, rotating the resultant current and allowing it to cover a larger area. This adjustment is called scanning on some equipment. There is little evidence that such adjustments are necessary.

In addition, some equipment provides a bipolar application of interferential current. These units are claimed to "mix the current in the machine." In actuality, the current produced is an amplitude-modulated medium frequency sine wave that can be applied with two pad electrodes.

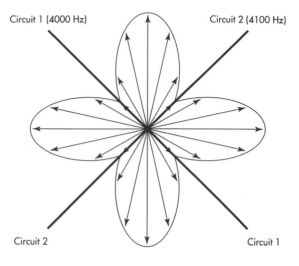

Circuit 1 (4000 Hz)

Circuit 2 (4100 Hz)

Circuit 2

Circuit 1

Figure 12–2. The interferential resultant current that is theoretically produced in a cloverleaf shape on a diagonal between the pathways of the two circuits.

PURPOSE AND EFFECTS

The effects of interferential current are consistent with those produced by other currents that provide the same phase duration (about 125 μsec) and frequency (1 to 100 beats per second) as the resultant current.

1. Using greater than 50 beats per second and low amplitudes, pain may be relieved by stimulating large afferent neurons and interfering with ascending (lemniscal) transmission of pain impulses.
2. Using 0 to 5 beats per second and an amplitude sufficient to produce muscle contractions may also relieve pain, but the mechanism of action is not known. The phase duration is too short to compare with those methods known to produce endogenous opioids or interfere with ascending (extralemniscal) transmission of pain impulses.
3. Frequencies of 0 to 10 beats per second produce small pulsating contractions of innervated muscle.
4. Frequencies of 30 to 50 beats per second produce tetanic contractions of innervated muscle. If used, the machine must also be able to modulate those contractions in some way. Because of the narrow phase duration, high intensities are necessary for muscle contractions, and interferential stimulation may not be effective in producing ample torque for muscle strengthening.[4]

ADVANTAGE

Because medium-frequency current faces low impedance as it crosses the skin, it may be able to target treatment sites slightly deeper than other types of electrical stimulation.

DISADVANTAGE

Even though the crossed paths are thought to target the site where they cross, current density still remains highest under the electrodes,[5] and the patient may not perceive much stimulation at the target site.

INDICATIONS

1. Pain relief.
2. Muscle exercise for increased blood flow, muscle relaxation, edema reduction,[6] and relief of urinary stress incontinence.[7-9]
3. Tissue and bone healing,[10] although this is disputed.[11]

CONTRAINDICATIONS

Please refer to those listed for electrical stimulation.

PRECAUTIONS

Please refer to those listed for electrical stimulation.

INSTRUCTIONS

1. Instruct the patient about the treatment and what you expect of her.
2. Check the patient's skin integrity and sensation.
3. Clean the skin and reduce skin impedance according to the instructions in the General Procedures for Electrical Stimulation in Chapter 10.
4. Position and drape the patient comfortably, allowing access to the part to be treated.
5. Determine the size and type of electrodes to use. Most units use pregelled self-adhesive disposable electrodes; others use silicon- or carbon-impregnated rubber electrodes that work with a film of water rather than conductive gel. Some older units use pad or suction electrodes with moistened sponge pads. *Note:* A small pad electrode with four conductive spots has been available with some machines. These electrodes should not be used because they create high current density and can cause burns.
6. Prepare electrodes depending on type. Pregelled electrodes may or may not need the application of a slight layer of moisture. Moisten the sponges for the pad electrodes with tap water, and attach them to the area to be treated using straps or sandbags. Suction electrodes are used very little, because they create erythematous patches on the skin. If they are used, place the electrodes on top of the machine to set the suction. Remove them by lifting the release valve (usually a small ring at the top) (Figure 12-3). Moisten the sponges and place them in the electrode cups. To apply the electrodes to the patient, squeeze the cup slightly, press it on the skin, and hold it for a few moments until the suction is established.
7. Attach the lead wires to the electrodes.
8. Apply the electrodes so that the current paths cross at the site of the problem. There are usually two red lead wires and two white lead wires to indicate the different circuits. In addition, the ends of the lead wires may also be color coded. If the machine has such coding, be sure that the lead wires that are closest together have the same color tips. This precaution is designed to help prevent skin currents.

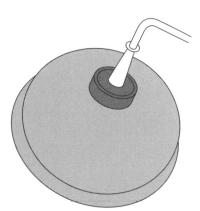

Figure 12-3. Vacuum (suction) electrodes previously used with interferential current. The gray ring is the vacuum release valve.

9. If using suction electrodes, adjust the suction to the least suction necessary to maintain adherence of the electrodes.

10. Select the appropriate frequency for the treatment goal. Decide whether the frequency is to be fixed or automatically swept and, if so, over what range.

11. Increase the amplitude of one circuit and then the other to a level appropriate for the goal. The patient should feel a sensation where the circuits cross at the target site.

12. Determine whether to use amplitude scanning. It is often used if the patient does not detect the stimulation sensation at the site or the site is difficult to determine.

13. Instruct the patient to keep movement to a minimum and to avoid handling the electrodes or the machine. Provide the patient with a call system.

14. Continue treatment for a time that is appropriate to reach the goal of treatment. If amplitude scanning is used, be aware that any area of tissue receives treatment for a shorter period of time, so an increase in the total treatment time is indicated.

15. At the end of the treatment, turn off the current. Remove the electrodes, turn off the machine, and dry the patient.

16. Perform all indicated posttreatment evaluations, including skin inspection.

17. Document the electrode placement, amplitude and frequencies used, whether amplitude scanning and/or frequency sweeping were used, duration of treatment, and the patient response.

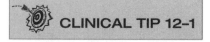

CLINICAL TIP 12-1

Targeting the Treatment Site

There is no best method to target the treatment site except trial and error. Rearranging the electrodes or altering the amplitude scanning may help locate the crossed current at the treatment site.

DOSAGE

Amplitude

The amplitude of treatment is determined by the goal of treatment. If interferential treatment is being used for pain relief, a sensory level is all that is necessary. Motor goals require higher intensities to achieve a muscle contraction.

Duration

Duration is also controlled by the goal of treatment, but a clinic-based treatment is usually 20 to 30 minutes.

Frequency

Frequency is controlled by the goal of treatment and may range from daily to two or three times per day.

RESPONSES TO TREATMENT AND TREATMENT MODIFICATION

The anticipated response to treatment is related to the goal. The patient should experience tingling both under the electrodes and in the target area where the currents from the two circuits cross. At the conclusion of treatment, the skin should show no changes in color or integrity. If treatment is ineffective, try rearranging the electrodes or using the amplitude scanning feature to target the site better. If the frequency sweep was not used, try using a range of frequencies; if it was used, try changing the range.

HOME USE

Portable interferential current generators are available for home use. These machines produce the amplitude-modulated medium frequency current that is used with the bipolar technique. If the patient responds well to clinical treatment, consider instructing her in renting and using one of these units.

REFERENCES

1. Lambert JL, Vanderstraeten GG, De Cuyper HJ, et al. Electric current distribution during interferential therapy. *Eur J Phys Med Rehabil.* 1993;3:6–10.
2. Deller AGM. Physical principles of interferential therapy. In: Savage B, ed. *Interferential Therapy.* London: Faber & Faber; 1984:15–26.
3. Johnson MI, Wilson H. The analgesic effects of different swing patterns of interferential currents on cold-induced pain. *Physiotherapy.* 1997;83:461–467.
4. Snyder-Mackler L, Garrett M, Roberts M. A comparison of torque generating capabilities of three different electrical stimulating currents. *J Orthop Sports Phys Ther.* 1989;10:297–301.
5. Treffene RJ. Interferential fields in a fluid medium. *Aust J Physiother.* 1983;29:209–216.
6. Ganne JM. Interferential therapy. *Aust J Physiother.* 1976;22:101–110.
7. Dougall DS. The effects of interferential therapy on incontinence and frequency of micturition. *Physiotherapy.* 1985;71:135–136.
8. Laycock J, Green RJ. Interferential therapy in the treatment of incontinence. *Physiotherapy.* 1988;74:161–168.
9. Laycock J, Jerwood D. Does pre-modulated interferential therapy cure genuine stress incontinence? *Physiotherapy.* 1993;79:553–560.
10. Ganne JM, Speculand B, Mayne LH, Goss AN. Interferential therapy to promote union of mandibular fractures. *Aust N Z J Surg.* 1979;49:81–83.
11. Taylor K, Newton RA, Personius WJ, Bush FM. Effects of interferential current stimulation for treatment of subjects with recurrent jaw pain. *Phys Ther.* 1987;67:346–350.

ADDITIONAL READINGS

DeDomenico G. *Basic Guidelines for Interferential Therapy.* Sydney, Australia: Theramed Books; 1981.

Nelson B. Interferential therapy. *Aust J Physiother.* 1981;27:53–56.

Proctor J, Casciato K, Finn L, et al. The effect of interferential current on finger temperature in patients with reflex sympathetic dystrophy [abstract]. *Physiother Can.* 1988; 40(2)(suppl):21.

Quirk AS, Newman RJ, Newman KJ. An evaluation of interferential therapy, shortwave diathermy and exercise in the treatment of osteoarthrosis of the knee. *Physiotherapy.* 1985;71:55–57.

Truscott B. Interferential therapy as a treatment for classical migraine: case reports. *Aust J Physiother.* 1984;30:33–35.

Willie CD. Interferential therapy. *Physiotherapy.* 1969;55:503–505.

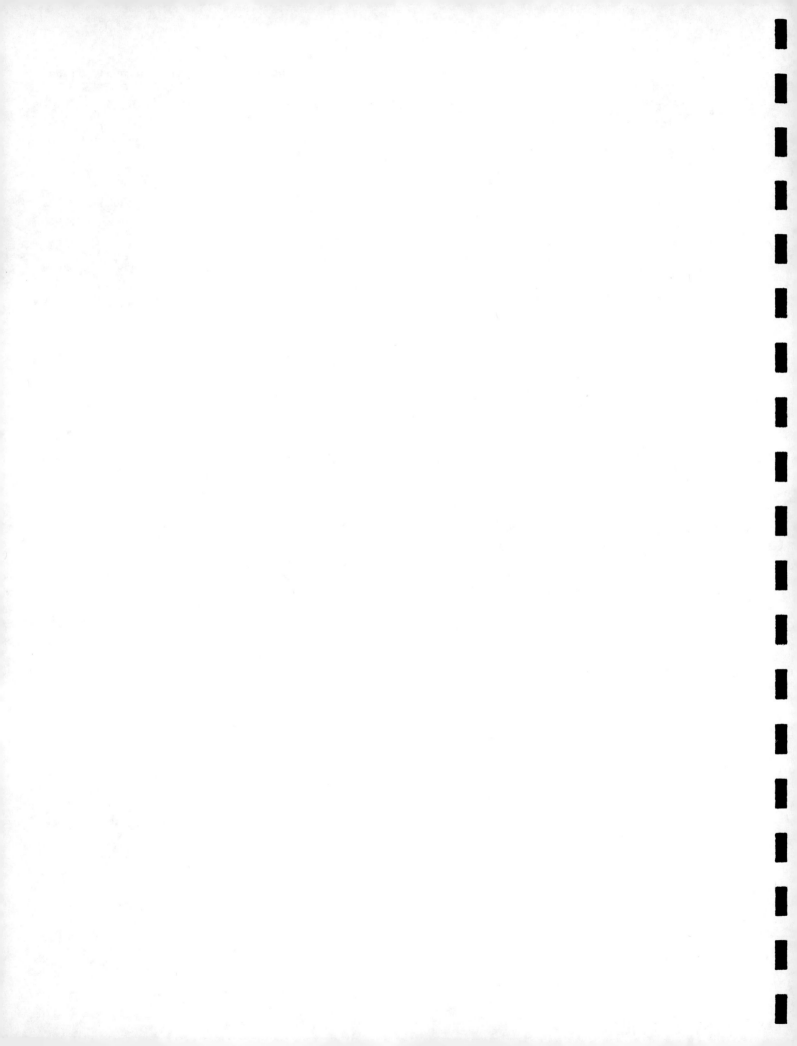

13

Iontophoresis

DESCRIPTION

Iontophoresis, or ion transfer, is the introduction of medicinal ions into the skin and mucous membranes of the body by the use of direct current. The principle on which it is based is the repulsion of the ion by the similarly charged electrode. The current and accompanying medication enter the skin through the pores associated with hair follicles and sweat glands. Ions are introduced using medicinal solutions or gels spread on the skin and covered with an electrode.

Direct current produces chemicals at both poles, altering the pH of the skin and potentially producing chemical burns, especially where the current is dense. Because of this risk, iontophoresis treatments are usually short, using low amplitudes of current. Recent research has shown that medications can be transferred and burns can be avoided by using long periods of low frequency alternating current.[1] More research concerning effectiveness, efficiency, and dosage is necessary before alternating current can be used on a routine basis.

PURPOSE AND EFFECTS

The purpose of ion transfer is to introduce medicinal ions locally, avoiding systemic distribution through the blood stream. The ions are deposited subcutaneously and are absorbed slowly, making prolonged treatment possible. The ions introduced have the same effects as they would have by any other means of introduction.

Penetration of the ions depends on several factors. The flow of direct current produces changes in pH that can affect the penetration of the ions.[2] Consequently, many electrode systems are buffered, both to allow predictable penetration of the ions and to protect the skin. Ions that are monovalent penetrate more easily than divalent ions.[2,3] Weak solutions allow easier penetration than stronger solutions.[4]

INDICATIONS

Historically, iontophoresis has been used for athlete's foot,[4] rhinitis,[5] slow healing wounds,[6,7] posttraumatic edema,[4,8] plantar warts,[9] trigger points,[4] rheumatoid arthritis,[4] peripheral circulatory deficits,[10,11] gout,[12] and myositis ossificans.[13] These uses are summarized in Table 13–1. While some of these applications are still occasionally used, the most common use for iontophoresis today is to treat inflammatory conditions of the musculoskeletal system with hydrocortisone or dexamethasone sodium phosphate with or without lidocaine hydrochloride. This treatment has been used successfully for epicondylitis,[14,15]

TABLE 13–1. Historical Uses of Iontophoresis

CONDITION	ION (POLARITY)	MODE OF ACTION	CONCENTRATION OF SOLUTION	DOSAGE
Athlete's foot[4]	Copper (+)	Fungicidal	1% copper sulfate solution	10 mA for 15 min; two times per week
Slow healing wounds[6]	Zinc (+)	Bactericidal	1.0 M zinc oxide gel (8.138 g zinc oxide powder, 10 g glycerol, 10 g bentonite, 71.862 g water)	3–6 mA for 20 min, increased to 25–30 min at end of each of first 2 weeks; 5 days a week for 3 weeks
Posttraumatic edema[4]	Hyaluronidase (+)	Breaks down hyaluronic acid	150 units of hyaluronidase in 250 mL of a buffer solution that consists of: (1) sodium acetate $3H_2O$: 11.42 g (2) Glacial acetic acid: 0.923 mL (3) Distilled H_2O, quantum satis (qs): 1000 mL	20 mA for 20 min; three times per week
Plantar warts[9]	Salicylate (–)	Removal and relief of pain	2% sodium salicylate in aqueous solution	10 mA●min; once per week for two or three treatments
Trigger points[4]	Procaine or lidocaine (+)	Local anesthesia (use with caution)	1% solution in 60–80% alcohol with 1:20,000 adrenalin	20–30 mA for 20–30 min; one to three times per day
Acute rheumatoid arthritis[4]	Citrate (–)	Prevents local autoimmune response	1% potassium citrate in distilled water	7.5–10 mA for 20 min; daily to three times per week
Peripheral circulatory deficit[10,11]	Histamine (+)	Vasodilator	1:10,000 histamine diphosphate	3–12 mA for 5 to 20 min (approximately 60 mA●min); two to three times per week
Gout[12]	Lithium (+)	Competes with sodium in formation of urate; lithium urate is soluble	2% lithium chloride	5 mA for 20 min; one time per week for 4 weeks
Myositis ossificans[13]	Acetate (–)	Absorption of calcium	3 mL of 2% acetic acid in distilled water	4 mA for 20 min; followed by ultrasound for 8 min at 1.5 W/cm^2 at 50% duty cycle

bursitis,[14] tendinitis,[14,16,17] myofascial syndrome,[18] rheumatoid arthritis,[19–21] plantar fasciitis,[22] and shinsplints.[23] The usual method of delivery of dexamethasone is included as an example in the Instructions section below.

CONTRAINDICATIONS

1. Anesthetic skin in the area to be treated. Be cautious if using local anesthetics as treatment (e.g., lidocaine, procaine, dibucaine).
2. Recent scars in the area to be treated.
3. Metal embedded close to the skin in the area to be treated.
4. Acute injury if active bleeding is still present.
5. Patients with cardiac pacemakers.

INSTRUCTIONS

1. Instruct the patient regarding what you are going to do, what to expect from treatment, and what you expect of him.
2. Clean the skin of oils, dry skin, and excess hair. Examine the skin and protect any open areas with cream, petroleum jelly, or waterproof tape. Check for skin sensation.
3. Prepare the medicinal solution or gel. Some preparations are commercially available, but it usually is necessary to work with a pharmacist to prepare an appropriate medium. One commonly used preparation for dexamethasone is 4 mg dexamethasone sodium phosphate in 1 mL sterile water with 2 mL of 4% lidocaine hydrochloride.

    In some states, physical therapists are not permitted by law to dispense medications, so the patient may need a prescription from the physician to obtain the preparation and bring it to the treatment.
4. Prepare the electrodes appropriately for the treatment to be given. Historically, pads or baths or a combination of both have been used depending on the area and condition to be treated. Modern equipment has now replaced these methods, allowing for better control of treatment dosage and skin pH.
    a. The electrodes that come with the modern systems are self-adherent. One type uses a gel-sponge pad that can be impregnated with the medicinal solution using an eyedropper or hypodermic syringe without the needle (Figure 13–1A). The other type of electrode has a pouch separated from the skin by a very fine, permeable membrane. The pouch is filled with medicinal solution using a hypodermic syringe (Figure 13–1B). Because of the risk of penetrating the membrane or the patient's skin with the syringe, the gel-sponges are becoming increasingly popular.
    b. These electrodes use different types of buffer systems to stabilize the pH of the solution to prevent skin damage and to ensure appropriate penetration of the drug.
    c. Use only enough solution to saturate the sponge; the solution should not ooze out around the electrode when it is attached.
5. Connect the leads to a direct current generator so that the polarity of the active electrode is the same as that of the ion to be introduced. For

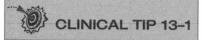

CLINICAL TIP 13–1

Drug Allergies

Some patients have known drug allergies and demonstrate the same symptoms whether the drug is taken orally, by injection, or through iontophoresis. Be sure to question the patient about drug allergies prior to treatment, and avoid using medications that are the same as or similar to those to which the patient is allergic. When in doubt about drug similarity, consult a pharmacist.

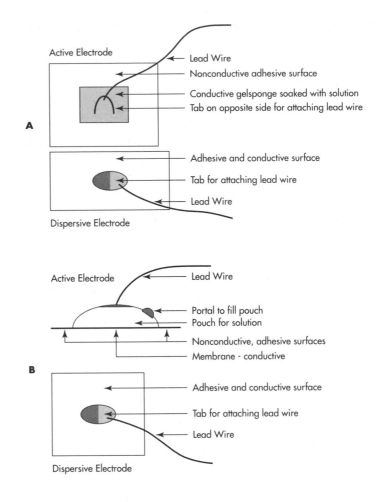

Figure 13–1. Commercial electrodes used in iontophoresis applications. A. Gelsponge electrode. B. Pouch electrode.

example, dexamethasone is a negative ion, so the negative electrode is used to introduce it. Attach the dispersive electrode to a convenient area of the skin nearby. The electrodes should be at least as far apart as the diameter of the larger electrode and preferably farther apart to prevent accidental arcing between the electrodes.

6. Position the patient appropriately and comfortably.

7. Apply the electrodes to the skin using tape or adhesive patches if the electrodes are not self-adherent. Be sure that self-adherent electrodes adhere well and reinforce them with tape if necessary.

8. Begin introducing continuous direct current slowly. *Never initiate, terminate, or interrupt the current abruptly.*

9. Dosage is based on the product of the current amplitude and the time for which it flows and is expressed in milliampere-minutes (mA•min). As long as the amplitude is within patient tolerance and the safety guide of 1 mA/in.^{2} (0.16 mA/cm^2) of the smaller electrode surface,[4] the amount of current and the time can be adjusted within the dosages suggested. For example, the usual dosage for dexamethasone iontophoresis is 80 mA•min. This dosage could be 4 mA for 20 minutes or 5 mA for 16 minutes.

Manufacturers of modern equipment have often set limits to the amount of amplitude that may be used during treatment. For example, the maximum amplitude may be set at 4 mA. This limitation is based on the maximum safe current density of 1 mA/in.^{2} (0.16 mA/cm^2) and an electrode size of 4 in.^{2} (26 cm^2).

10. Terminate the treatment by slowly returning the amplitude to zero and giving appropriate follow-up care.
11. Perform all indicated posttreatment evaluations, including a skin inspection.
12. Document the medication and preparation used, location of the electrodes, dosage given, duration of treatment, and patient response.

DOSAGE

Please refer to the specific techniques listed in Table 13–1. Treatment with dexamethasone is usually given daily.

RESPONSES TO TREATMENT

Because continuous direct current is used in iontophoresis, chemical reactions take place at both electrodes, especially if buffered electrode systems are not used. As a result, the skin is pink under both electrodes, especially the cathode, following treatment. Pink skin is a normal response; however, very red skin with swelling may indicate a burn. If the patient has very dark skin, changes in skin color may not be observed. Burns are more common at the cathode due to the alkaline change in pH.

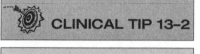

CLINICAL TIP 13–2

Electrode Size

Because the skin reaction is often stronger at the cathode, the intensity of the reaction may be decreased by decreasing the current density under the cathode. Make the cathode at least twice as large as the anode, regardless of the polarity of the ion being introduced.

HOME USE

Although the units used to deliver iontophoresis are portable, the hazard associated with the use of direct current and medication are such that iontophoresis should not be used as a home treatment.

REFERENCES

1. Howard JP, Drake TR, Kellogg DL. Effects of alternating current iontophoresis on drug delivery. *Arch Phys Med Rehabil.* 1995;76:463–466.
2. Costello CT, Jeske AH. Iontophoresis: applications in transdermal medication delivery. *Phys Ther.* 1995;75:554–563.
3. Li LC, Scudds RA. Iontophoresis: an overview of the mechanisms and clinical application. *Arthritis Care Res.* 1995;8:51–61.
4. Harris R. Iontophoresis. In: Licht S, ed. *Therapeutic Electricity and Ultraviolet Radiation.* 2nd ed. Baltimore: Williams & Wilkins; 1967:156–178.
5. Rady DJ. Zinc ionization as a treatment for chronic rhinitis. *Aust J Physiother.* 1972;18:148–150.
6. Balogun JA, Abidoye AB, Akala EO. Zinc iontophoresis in the management of bacterial colonized wounds: a case report. *Physiother Can.* 1990;42:147–151.
7. Cornwall MW. Zinc iontophoresis to treat ischemic skin ulcers. *Phys Ther.* 1981;61:359–360.

8. Magistro CM. Hyaluronidase by iontophoresis. *Phys Ther.* 1964;44:169–175.
9. Gordon AH, Weinstein MV. Sodium salicylate iontophoresis in the treatment of plantar warts. *Phys Ther.* 1969;49:869–870.
10. Abramson DI, Tuck S, Chu LS, Buso E. Physiologic and clinical basis for histamine by ion transfer. *Arch Phys Med Rehabil.* 1967;48:583–591.
11. Abramson DI, Tuck S, Zayas AM, et al. Vascular responses produced by histamine by ion transfer. *J Appl Physiol.* 1963;18:305–310.
12. Kahn J. A case report: lithium iontophoresis for gouty arthritis. *J Orthop Sports Phys Ther.* 1982;4:113–114.
13. Weider DL. Treatment of traumatic myositis ossificans with acetic acid iontophoresis. *Phys Ther.* 1992;72:133–137.
14. Harris PR. Iontophoresis: clinical research in musculoskeletal inflammatory conditions. *J Orthop Sports Phys Ther.* 1982;4:109–112.
15. Panus PC, Hooper T, Padrones A, et al. A case study of exacerbation of lateral epicondylitis by combined use of iontophoresis and phonophoresis. *Physiother Can.* 1996;48:27–31.
16. Pellecchia GL, Hamel H, Behnke P. Treatment of infrapatellar tendinitis: a combination of modalities and transverse friction massage versus iontophoresis. *J Sport Rehabil.* 1994;3:135–145.
17. Bertolucci LE. Introduction of antiinflammatory drugs by iontophoresis: double blind study. *J Orthop Sports Phys Ther.* 1982;4:103–108.
18. DeLacerda FG. A comparative study of three methods of treatment for shoulder girdle myofascial syndrome. *J Orthop Sports Phys Ther.* 1982;4:51–54.
19. Hasson SH, Henderson GH, Daniels JC, Schieb DA. Exercise training and dexamethasone iontophoresis in rheumatoid arthritis: a case study. *Physiother Can.* 1991;43:11–14, 29.
20. Hasson SM, English SE, Daniels JC, Reich M. Effect of iontophoretically delivered dexamethasone on muscle performance in a rheumatoid arthritic joint: a case study. *Arthritis Care Res.* 1988;1:177–182.
21. Li LC, Scudds RA, Heck CS, Harth M. The efficacy of dexamethasone iontophoresis for the treatment of rheumatoid arthritic knees: a pilot study. *Arthritis Care Res.* 1996;9:126–132.
22. Gudeman SD, Eisele SA, Heidt RS, et al. Treatment of plantar fasciitis by iontophoresis of 0.4% dexamethasone: a randomized, double-blind, placebo-controlled study. *Am J Sports Med.* 1997;25:312–316.
23. DeLacerda FG. Iontophoresis for treatment of shinsplints. *J Orthop Sports Phys Ther.* 1981;3:183–185.

ADDITIONAL READINGS

Boone DC. Applications of iontophoresis. In: Wolf SL, ed. *Electrotherapy.* New York: Churchill Livingstone; 1981:99–121.

Downer AH. Treatment of acute torticollis with ion transfer. *Phys Ther Rev.* 1956;36:321–322.

Garzione JE. Salicylate iontophoresis as an alternative treatment for persistent thigh pain following hip surgery. *Phys Ther.* 1978;58:570–571.

Glass JM, Stephen RC, Jacobson SC. The quantity and distribution of radiolabeled dexamethasone delivered to tissue by iontophoresis. *Int J Dermatol.* 1980;19:519–525.

Kahn J. Calcium iontophoresis in suspected myopathy. *Phys Ther.* 1975;55:376–377.

Kahn J. Non-steroid iontophoresis. *Clin Manage Phys Ther.* 1987;7(1):14–15.

Kahn J. Use of iontophoresis in Peyronie's disease. *Phys Ther.* 1982;62:995–996.

Langley PL. Iontophoresis to aid in releasing tendon adhesions. *Phys Ther.* 1984;64:1395.

Perron M, Malouin F. Acetic acid iontophoresis and ultrasound for the treatment of calcifying tendinitis of the shoulder: a randomized control trial. *Arch Phys Med Rehabil.* 1997;78:379–384.

Puttemans FJM, Massart D, Gilles F, et al. Iontophoresis: mechanism of action studied by potentiometry and x-ray fluorescence. *Arch Phys Med Rehabil.* 1982;63:176–180.

Stralka SW, Head PL, Mohr K. The clinical use of iontophoresis. *Phys Ther Prod.* 1996;7(2):48–51.

Zankel HT. Effect of physical modalities upon Ra^{131} iontophoresis. *Arch Phys Med Rehabil.* 1963;44:93–97.

chapter 14

High-Voltage Pulsed Current

DESCRIPTION

High-voltage pulsed current (HVPC) is another means of delivering electrical stimuli to accomplish a variety of therapeutic purposes. The two major differences between HVPC and other types of stimulation are the waveform of the current and the voltage of the generator. The waveform of HVPC (Figure 14–1) consists of paired, unidirectional impulses that rise instantaneously and decay exponentially. The phase duration at the base of each member of a pair is 50 to 100 µsec but is much less as the peak of the spike is approached. Some HVPC units are capable of altering the space between the members of each pair of pulses. The phase duration is insufficient to stimulate denervated muscle, and the units are unsatisfactory for performing iontophoresis. The exceptionally narrow phase duration of the wave form used in HVPC is the reason high voltages are necessary. High-voltage units have an electromotive force of up to 500 volts. Other stimulators usually do not exceed 150 volts. Higher voltages bypass the impedance of the skin, allowing use of lower current amplitudes in patient treatment.[1]

The units that provide HVPC allow the use of a handheld applicator (Figure 14–2A) or pad electrodes. Two or four pad electrodes may be attached to the active lead wire, and all are of the same polarity. A large dispersive electrode of the opposite polarity is used to complete the circuit (Figure 14–2B and C). The dispersive electrode provided with these units is very large so that it is larger than the combined areas of four of the pad electrodes. Alternatively, one pad may be attached to the active lead wire, and the other pad can be attached to the dispersive lead wire to produce a bipolar application (Figure 14–2D).

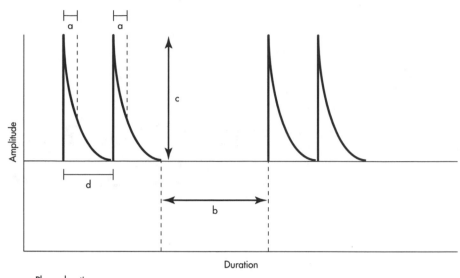

a. Phase duration
b. Interpulse interval
c. Peak amplitude
d. Phase separation

Figure 14–1. Waveform produced by high-voltage pulsed current stimulators. A. Phase duration. B. Interpulse interval. C. Peak amplitude. D. Phase separation.

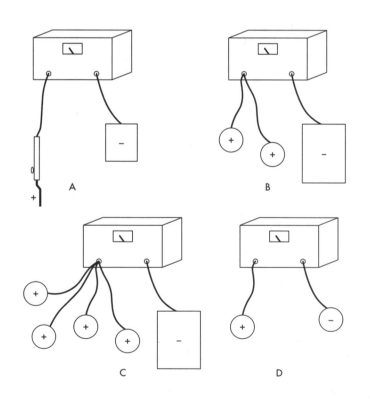

Figure 14–2. Configurations of electrodes used with high-voltage pulsed current. A. Handheld applicator. B. Two active pads, both of the same polarity (+). C. Four active pads, both of the same polarity (+). D. Bipolar with two pads, one positive and one negative. The large dispersive pad is not used.

PURPOSE AND EFFECTS

In that HVPC is electrical stimulation, the effects are similar to those already discussed with other modes of stimulation.

1. The frequency, phase duration, and amplitude ranges of HVPC are appropriate to stimulate the large afferent neurons selectively. Stimulation of the A beta neurons has been proposed to promote pain relief through the spinal gating mechanism.[2]
2. Pain may be relieved through relief of muscle guarding. As a muscle stimulator, HVPC can produce an intermittent contraction to promote blood flow and produce relaxation.
3. Edema may be curbed or reduced using the possible polar effects of HVPC.[3–6] Following acute injury, proteins escape from the microvasculature. Cathodal stimulation can repel these proteins from the area, taking excess fluid with them.[7]
4. As a muscle stimulator, HVPC can be used for muscle exercise for a variety of goals such as preventing disuse atrophy, improving blood flow, or reeducation. Because the phase duration is so narrow, HVPC may not be as efficient a muscle stimulator as one that produces a longer stimulus duration.
5. Through possible polar effects, HVPC can promote accelerated tissue healing.[8,9] Naturally occurring bioelectric currents are enhanced, increasing phagocytosis, contraction, and epithelialization in moist, clean wounds.[10] Cathodal stimulation has been shown to be bactericidal,[11] whereas anodal stimulation may attract fibroblasts and neutrophils.[12,13] Wound care with HVPC has been shown to be cost effective.[14]

INDICATIONS

In addition to enhancing motor performance (Chapter 10) and pain reduction (Chapter 11), HVPC can serve two goals:

1. Promote wound healing.
2. Curb or reduce edema, especially acute edema.

CONTRAINDICATIONS AND PRECAUTIONS

HVPC is another form of electrical stimulation. The contraindications and precautions are the same as those previously listed for other modes of electrical stimulation.

INSTRUCTIONS

1. Instruct the patient about what to expect and what you expect of her.
2. Position and drape the patient appropriately, allowing accessibility of the skin surfaces where electrodes will be placed.
3. Check the patient's skin for integrity and sensation.
4. Clean the skin and reduce skin impedance (see general instructions for using electrical stimulators).

5. Prepare the dispersive electrode (see general instructions for using electrical stimulators), and position it on the same body surface at some distance away. The size of the dispersive electrode provided with these units requires a large body surface such as the back, abdomen, or thigh.

6. Prepare either the handheld applicator or pads. If the electrodes are the sponge type, wet the sponges and place them over the electrodes. Cover the sponges with clean, wet gauze. Some electrodes have no sponges and require only a thin film of water. If treating a wound, use fluffed-up sterile gauze rather than the sponge electrodes and normal saline solution rather than water.[10]

7. If using the pads, position them firmly over the involved area. Secure them with straps, sandbags, or by body weight.

8. The handheld applicator may be used by holding it firmly over the involved area or by gently sliding it around the involved area, maintaining firm contact. The handheld applicator on many clinical stimulators has a separate amplitude control on the applicator.

9. Select the polarity, frequency, and mode appropriate for the problem. If using HVPC for motor goals, the active electrode should be negative to depolarize the alpha motor neurons. For pain reduction, there is no evidence that suggests a preference of one polarity over the other for the active electrode.

10. Turn the unit on and turn the amplitude up to the sensory or motor level appropriate for the treatment goal.

11. Allow sufficient treatment time to accomplish the goal of treatment.

12. To terminate the treatment, return the intensity to zero. Remove the equipment, and dry the patient. Dress any wounds that are present. Clean the sponges with a disinfectant such as povidone-iodine and rinse thoroughly.

13. Perform all appropriate posttreatment evaluations, including a skin inspection.

14. Document the goal of treatment, mode used, arrangement of electrodes, frequency, amplitude, duration of treatment, and all patient responses.

Underwater Treatment Instructions

This treatment is for uneven or tender surfaces.

1. Prepare the patient as above.
2. Fill a fiberglass or plastic pan with warm water to a depth sufficient to cover the involved area.
3. Place the pad electrodes without the sponges into the pan in such a way that they *cannot* contact the patient.
4. Remove the clothing from the part to be treated, position the patient comfortably, and immerse the involved part.
5. Place the dispersive electrode under the back, abdomen, buttock, or thigh. Secure with straps or body weight. The surface area of the skin that is in actual contact with the water constitutes the active electrode.

CLINICAL TIP 14–1

Polarity and Frequency for Wound Healing

In general, use the highest frequency the HVPC unit provides to maximize the transfer of electrical charge to the patient. The amplitude has to be submotor to prevent a prolonged contraction. In clean wounds, use the positive electrode as the active electrode to enhance epithelialization and autolytic débridement. For infected or inflamed wounds, use the negative electrode as the active electrode to attract neutrophils, kill bacteria,[11] and promote granulation.[10]

Because this area is likely to be substantial, it may prove necessary to increase the size of the dispersive electrode to prevent the patient from experiencing a response under it. To do so, place a folded, wet towel over the electrode and in contact with the skin.

6. Increase the amplitude to the sensory or motor level appropriate for the treatment goal. Allow sufficient time to accomplish the goal.
7. To terminate the treatment, return the intensity to zero and remove the equipment. Dry the skin and dress any wounds present. Clean the electrodes and the pan with a disinfectant.
8. Perform all indicated posttreatment evaluations, including a skin inspection.
9. Document the goal of treatment, mode used, arrangement of electrodes, frequency, amplitude, duration of treatment, and all patient responses.

RESPONSES TO TREATMENT AND TREATMENT MODIFICATION

Depending on the goal, the patient should experience only a sensation of tingling or a motor response. The narrow phase duration of HVPC makes response from pain fibers unlikely, but if the patient experiences pain, respond by decreasing the amplitude and allowing the patient more time to adjust to the treatment.

DOSAGE

Intensity
For motor and pain goals, follow the guidelines given in Chapters 10 and 11.

Duration
The dosage depends on the goal. For motor and pain goals, see the guidelines given in Chapters 10 and 11.

Frequency
The frequency is determined by the goal. Pain reduction and exercise treatments may be performed daily or twice daily. Treatment for edema and wound healing may be done up to four times a day.

HOME USE

Small, portable units that produce HVPC are available. If the patient would benefit from use of stimulation more frequently than can be provided in the clinical setting, procure a unit and instruct the patient regarding its use. Be sure to include information regarding electrode placement, polarity, frequency, amplitude, and duration of treatment. Many vendors allow patients to rent units for a finite period of time.

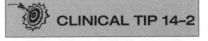
CLINICAL TIP 14–2

Dosage for Wound Healing

To be effective in wound healing, treatment must be given for at least 60 minutes per day, 5 days per week.[10]

REFERENCES

1. Mueller EE, Loeffel R, Mead S. Skin impedance in relation to pain threshold testing by electrical means. *J Appl Physiol.* 1952;5:746–752.
2. Melzack R, Wall PD. Pain mechanisms: a new theory. *Science.* 1965;150:971–979.
3. Bettany JA, Fish DR, Mendel FC. Influence of high voltage pulsed direct current on edema formation following impact injury. *Phys Ther.* 1990;70:219–224.
4. Fish DR, Mendel FC, Schultz AM, Gottstein-Yerka LM. Effect of anodal high voltage pulsed current on edema formation in frog hind limbs. *Phys Ther.* 1991;71:724–733.
5. Taylor K, Fish DR, Mendel FC, Burton HW. Effect of a single 30-minute treatment of high voltage pulsed current on edema formation in frog hind limbs. *Phys Ther.* 1992;72:63–68.
6. Griffin JW, Tooms RE, Mendius RA, et al. Efficacy of high voltage pulsed current for healing of pressure ulcers in patients with spinal cord injury. *Phys Ther.* 1991;71:433–444.
7. Reed BV. Effect of high voltage pulsed electrical stimulation on microvascular permeability to plasma proteins: a possible mechanism in minimizing edema. *Phys Ther.* 1988;68:491–495.
8. Brown M, McDonnell MK, Menton DN. Polarity effects on wound healing using electric stimulation in rabbits. *Arch Phys Med Rehabil.* 1989;70:624–627.
9. Kloth LC, Feedar JA. Acceleration of wound healing with high voltage, monophasic, pulsed current. *Phys Ther.* 1988;68:503–598.
10. Kloth LC. Physical modalities in wound management: UVC, therapeutic heating and electrical stimulation. *Ostomy/Wound Manage.* 1995;41(5):18–20, 22–24, 26–27.
11. Kincaid CB, Lavoie KH. Inhibition of bacterial growth in vitro following stimulation with high voltage, monophasic, pulsed current. *Phys Ther.* 1989;69:651–655.
12. Feedar JA, Kloth LC, Gentzkow GD. Chronic dermal ulcer healing enhanced with monophasic pulsed electrical stimulation. *Phys Ther.* 1991;71:639–649.
13. Wolcott L, Wheeler P, Hardwicke H, Rowley B. Accelerated healing of skin ulcers by electrotherapy: preliminary clinical results. *South Med J.* 1969;62:795–801.
14. Swanson GH. Use of cost data, provider experience, and clinical guidelines in the transition to managed care. *J Insur Med.* 1991;23:70–74.

ADDITIONAL READINGS

Alon G. High voltage stimulation: effects of electrode size on basic excitatory responses. *Phys Ther.* 1985;65:890–895.

Alon G, Bainbridge J, Croson G, et al. High voltage pulsed direct current effects on peripheral blood flow [abstract R-176]. *Phys Ther.* 1981;61:734.

Brown M, Gogia PP. Effects of high voltage stimulation on cutaneous wound healing in rabbits. *Phys Ther.* 1987;67:662–667.

Brown M, McDonnell MK, Menton DN. Electrical stimulation effects on cutaneous wound healing in rabbits: a follow-up study. *Phys Ther.* 1988;68:955–960.

Brown S. Ankle edema and galvanic muscle stimulation. *Phys Sportsmed.* 1981;9:137.

Carley PJ, Wainapel SF. Electrotherapy for acceleration of wound healing: low intensity direct current. *Arch Phys Med Rehabil.* 1985;66:443–446.

Clemente FR, Malulionis DH, Barron KW, Currier DP. Effect of motor neuromuscular electrical stimulation on microvascular perfusion of stimulated rat skeletal muscle. *Phys Ther.* 1991;71:397–406.

Cosgrove KA, Alon G, Bell SF, et al. The electrical effect of two commonly used clinical stimulators on traumatic edema in rats. *Phys Ther.* 1992;72:227–233.

Fitzgerald GK, Newsome D. Treatment of a large infected thoracic spine wound using high voltage pulsed monophasic current. *Phys Ther.* 1993;73:355–360.

Gault WR, Gatens PF. Use of low intensity direct current in management of ischemic skin ulcers. *Phys Ther.* 1976;56:265–269.

Griffin JW, Newsome LS, Stralka SW, Wright PE. Reduction of chronic posttraumatic hand edema: a comparison of high voltage pulsed current, intermittent pneumatic compression, and placebo treatments. *Phys Ther*. 1990;70:279–286.

Guffey JS, Asmussen MD. In vitro bactericidal effects of high voltage pulsed current versus direct current against *Staphylococcus aureus. J Clin Electrophysiol*. 1989;1(1):5–9.

Hecker B, Carron H, Schwartz DP. Pulsed galvanic stimulation: effects of current frequency and polarity on blood flow in healthy subjects. *Arch Phys Med Rehabil*. 1985;66: 369–371.

Kalinowski DP, Brogan MS, Sleeper MD. A practical technique for disinfecting electrical stimulation apparatuses used in wound treatment. *Phys Ther*. 1996;76:1340–1347.

Karnes JL, Mendel FC, Fish DR. Effects of low voltage pulsed current on edema formation in frog hind limbs following impact injury. *Phys Ther*. 1992;72:273–278.

Kolb P, Denegar C. Traumatic edema and the lymphatic system. *Athletic Training*. 1983;17:339–341.

McMeeken J. Tissue temperature and blood flow: a research based overview of electrophysical modalities. *Aust J Physiother*. 1994;40(4):49–57.

Mendel FC, Wylegala JA, Fish DR. Influence of high voltage pulsed current on edema formation following impact injury in rats. *Phys Ther* 1992;72:668–673.

Michlovitz A, Smith W, Watkins M. Ice and high voltage pulsed stimulation in treatment of acute lateral ankle sprains. *J Orthop Sports Phys Ther*. 1988;9:301–304.

Mohr T, Akers TK, Landry R. Effect of high voltage stimulation on edema reduction in the rat hind limb. *Phys Ther*. 1987;67:1703–1707.

Mohr T, Akers TK, Wessman HC. Effects of high voltage stimulation on blood flow in the rat hind limb. *Phys Ther*. 1987;67:526–533.

Mohr T, Carlson B, Sulentis C, Landry R. Comparison of isometric exercise and high volt galvanic stimulation on quadriceps femoris muscle strength. *Phys Ther*. 1985;65:606–612.

Mohr T, Danzl L, Akers TK, Landry R. The effect of high volt galvanic stimulation on quadriceps femoris muscle torque. *J Orthop Sports Phys Ther*. 1986;7:314–318.

Newton RA, Karselis TC. Skin pH following high voltage pulsed galvanic stimulation. *Phys Ther*. 1983;63:1593–1596.

Quirion-deGirardi C, Seaborne D, Savard-Goulet FW, et al. The analgesic effect of high voltage galvanic stimulation combined with ultrasound in the treatment of low back pain: a one-group pretest/post-test study. *Physiother Can*. 1984;36:327–333.

Rosendal T. Studies on the conducting properties of the human skin to direct current. *Acta Physiol Scand*. 1943;5:130–151.

Sohn N, Weinstein MA, Robbins RD. The levator syndrome and its treatment with high voltage electrogalvanic stimulation. *Am J Surg*. 1982;144:580–582.

Szuminsky NJ, Albers AC, Unger P, Eddy JG. Effect of narrow, pulsed high voltages on bacterial viability. *Phys Ther*. 1994;74:660–667.

Thornton RM, Mendel FC, Fish DR. Effects of electrical stimulation on edema formation in different strains of rats. *Phys Ther*. 1998;78:386–394.

Thurman BF, Christian EL. Response of a serious circulatory lesion to electrical stimulation. *Phys Ther*. 1971;51:1107–1110.

Walker DC, Currier DP, Threlkeld AJ. Effects of high voltage pulsed electrical stimulation on blood flow. *Phys Ther*. 1988;68:481–485.

Wasson LC, Wasson SD. Electrical potentials and tissue regeneration. *J Clin Eng*. 1979;4:39–43.

Wheeler P, Wolcott L, Morris J, Spangler M. Neural considerations in the healing of ulcerated tissue by clinical electrotherapeutic application of weak direct current: findings and theory. In: Reynolds DF, ed. *Neuroelectric Research*. Springfield, Ill: Charles C Thomas; 1969:83–99.

Wong RA. High voltage versus low voltage electrical stimulation: force of induced muscle contraction and perceived discomfort in healthy subjects. *Phys Ther*. 1986;66:1209–1214.

Electrophysiologic Evaluation

*E*lectrophysiologic evaluation involves the use of stimulating currents on nerve, muscle, or both tissues for the purpose of aiding in the diagnosis and prognosis of sensorimotor deficits and for gathering data for treatment planning, monitoring patient status, or research. Precision in the performance of electrophysiologic measurements is important. To produce results that have meaning, all tests should be performed serially and should include data gathered from the contralateral muscle. To provide accuracy and consistency, the following guidelines should be considered in performing tests:

1. Select a test muscle that is innervated solely by the nerve to be tested and that is easily located and identified.
2. Try to maintain skin impedance at the same level for each test. Be consistent with procedures used to reduce impedance and test at the same point in the treatment plan each time. The following factors affect skin impedance:
   a. Moist heat prior to testing decreases skin impedance.
   b. Compression or restrictive garments increase skin impedance.
   c. Edema in the area to be tested increases impedance.
   d. Exercise prior to testing decreases impedance.
3. Select the same size and type of electrodes, prepare them in the same manner, and place them in the same location for each test.
4. Except for nerve conduction velocity testing, use minimal visible contractions as the testing index. They are easier to reproduce consistently than other indices and provide a means of confirming which muscle is being stimulated.
5. Even though the motor point disappears when the muscle is denervated, to provide an accurate index of progress over time, perform tests with the active electrode proximal on the muscle belly in the area where the motor point would normally be located.

6. If a test involves using direct current, use the cathode as the stimulating electrode.

Reaction of Degeneration

DESCRIPTION

The reaction of degeneration (RD) test, an historical test that is no longer used clinically to make decisions about patient status, is a simple, classic qualitative test that is quickly performed. It is included here as a teaching tool to aid in the understanding of the physiologic responses of nerve and muscle to various electrical stimuli. Having this understanding helps the practitioner explain unanticipated patient responses and may be instrumental in identifying a nerve lesion that is worse than it appears. The test is based on the differences between the reactions of innervated and denervated muscles to short and long duration stimuli.

PURPOSE

The RD test can help determine the integrity of the nerve–muscle complex and give a crude indication of whether denervation is complete.

ADVANTAGE

The RD test is easily performed and can provide a very quick indication of the integrity of the nerve–muscle complex.

DISADVANTAGES

1. The RD test is qualitative and subjective in nature.
2. The test can provide false information if the operator is imprecise or has not gathered appropriate data from the patient interview and other physical examinations.

INDICATIONS

1. The RD test can be used to aid in determining whether a peripheral nerve is intact, partially damaged, or completely interrupted.
2. The test can serve as an aid in distinguishing paralysis associated with an upper motor neuron lesion or hysteria from that associated with a lower motor neuron lesion.

CONTRAINDICATIONS

1. Because the RD test is performed with electrical stimulation, all contraindications and precautions listed for other modes of electrical stimulation must be observed.
2. The test is not valid if the muscle has been diseased or damaged.

INSTRUCTIONS

1. Instruct the patient regarding what to expect from the procedure and what you expect of him.
2. Check the area to be tested for skin sensation and integrity.
3. Select an electrical generator that allows a choice of long or short duration stimuli.
4. Test the uninvolved side first to provide a basis for comparison.
5. Test with short-duration stimuli. Perform the RD test on the involved nerve and at least two muscles innervated exclusively by that nerve, one proximal and one distal within the distribution of the nerve. The nerve can also be tested at several sites along its course to help determine approximately where in its course it is involved. For example, test the ulnar nerve at the elbow and at the wrist; test the flexor carpi ulnaris and the abductor digiti minimi. Sites of nerve testing and the muscles selected must relate to the history of the patient's complaints and pertinent physical findings (e.g., motor and sensory deficits).

   a. Set up the generator for a tetanizing current. The phase duration must be less than 1 msec and the frequency high enough to tetanize normal muscle. If a continuous sine or square wave alternating current is used, at least 500 Hz is necessary. If a symmetric or asymmetric biphasic pulsed current is used, any tetanizing frequency is adequate.

   b. Prepare and apply a dispersive electrode to an appropriate area (see general instructions for using electrical stimulation).

   c. Prepare the electrode, and connect it to the generator. The actual test was performed with an electrode handle with an interruptor switch and a small disc electrode. Today, a small pad electrode is more available and can be used.

   d. Locate the motor point of the nerve or muscle to be tested by increasing the current amplitude until a contraction occurs. When stimulating a nerve, the practitioner monitors the response in a distal reference muscle innervated by that nerve. When stimulating a muscle, the practitioner monitors the response in that muscle. Try to obtain a good strong contraction. It may be necessary to reposition the electrode until the best response is located.

   e. Note the quality of the contraction and record it (e.g., brisk, vermicular [wormy], smaller than uninvolved side, no response). Decrease the amplitude until a minimal visible contraction is obtained. Record the amplitude in Figure 15–1.

Patient:			Examiner:			Nerve tested:
Date	Test Site	Response to short duration stimulus		Response to long duration stimulus		Interpretation (N, PRD, FRD, ARD)*
		Right (mA)	Left (mA)	Right (mA)	Left (mA)	

*N = normal; PRD = partial reaction of degeneration; FRD = full reaction of degeneration; ARD = absolute reaction of degeneration

Figure 15–1. Recording form for reaction of degeneration test.

    f. Return the amplitude to zero.

    g. Do NOT remove the active electrode from the motor point.

6. Test with long duration stimuli.

    a. Change the current to a long-duration stimulus. A long-duration stimulus must be at least 100 msec. Traditionally, manually interrupted direct current was chosen because it was available on many generators, and the stimulus duration is about 500 msec.

    b. If using direct current, make the dispersive electrode positive and the active electrode negative. The active electrode should still be on the motor point.

    c. If using an electrode with an interruptor switch, interrupt the circuit rhythmically, increasing the amplitude until a contraction is observed. Record the quality of the contraction.

    d. Decrease the amplitude until a minimal visible contraction is obtained.

    e. Record the milliammeter reading.

    f. Reduce the amplitude to zero.

7. Repeat steps 5 and 6 for each nerve or muscle tested.

8. Determine the same data for the involved side.

9. Remove the equipment, and dry the patient. Check the patient's skin and general physiologic responses.

10. Document the current used, stimulation sites, and patient responses to all stimulation.

RESPONSES TO TESTING AND THEIR INTERPRETATION

The response to stimulation depends on the status of the nerve–muscle complex (type of injury), whether the injury is complete or incomplete, the site of stimulation, and the duration of the stimulus. Table 15–1 summarizes typical responses of nerve and muscle tissue in different states of nerve–muscle complex integrity.

TABLE 15–1. Interpretation of Results of Reaction of Degeneration Test

CONDITION AND STIMULATION SITE	RESPONSE TO SHORT-DURATION TETANIZING STIMULUS	RESPONSE TO LONG-DURATION SINGLE STIMULUS
Normal		
Nerve stimulated anywhere along its course	Tetanic contraction in all muscles innervated by that nerve distal to site of stimulation	Brisk twitch in all muscles innervated by that nerve distal to site of stimulation
Muscle stimulated directly	Tetanic contraction in that muscle	Brisk twitch in that muscle
Complete neurapraxia (conduction block) or axonotmesis or neurotmesis (axonal degeneration) in first day or two		
Nerve stimulated above site of block or lesion	No response in distal musculature innervated by nerve	No response in distal musculature innervated by nerve
Nerve stimulated below site of block or lesion	Normal tetanic contraction—nerve is conducting below block or lesion	Brisk twitch in muscles innervated distally to site of stimulation—nerve is conducting below block or lesion
Muscle above or below site of block or lesion	Normal tetanic contraction—nerve is conducting at site of stimulation	Brisk twitch—nerve is conducting at site of stimulation
Incomplete neurapraxia (conduction block) or axonotmesis or neurotmesis (axonal degeneration) in first day or two		
Nerve stimulated above site of block or lesion	Some response in distal musculature innervated by nerve—it is normal appearing but smaller than opposite side	Some response in distal musculature innervated by nerve—it is normal appearing but smaller than opposite side
Nerve stimulated below site of block or lesion	Normal tetanic contraction—nerve is conducting below block or lesion	Brisk twitch in muscles innervated distally to site of stimulation—nerve is conducting below block or lesion
Muscle above or below site of block or lesion	Normal tetanic contraction—nerve is conducting at site of stimulation	Brisk twitch—nerve is conducting at site of stimulation
Complete axonotmesis or neurotmesis after 14 days (full reaction of degeneration)		
Nerve stimulated above site of lesion	No response in distal musculature innervated by nerve	No response in distal musculature innervated by nerve
Nerve stimulated below site of lesion	No response in distal musculature innervated by nerve	No response in distal musculature innervated by nerve
Muscle stimulated below site of lesion	No response	Vermicular contraction—muscle is being stimulated directly
Incomplete axonotmesis or neurotmesis after 14 days (partial reaction of degeneration)		
Nerve stimulated above site of lesion	Diminished tetanic response in any or all of muscles innervated by that nerve distal to stimulation site	Diminished twitch response in any or all muscles innervated by that nerve distal to stimulation site
Nerve stimulated below site of lesion	Diminished tetanic response in any or all of muscles innervated by that nerve distal to stimulation site	Diminished twitch response in any or all muscles innervated by that nerve distal to stimulation site
Muscle stimulated below site of lesion	Diminished tetanic response compared to opposite side	Diminished twitch or vermicular response or both, depending on severity of lesion

1. The presence of the reaction of degeneration usually indicates denervation. If there is no response to either short- or long-duration stimuli, the response is labeled an absolute RD. The absolute RD indicates loss of muscle tissue as well and would be seen in injuries of long standing. No response to either stimulus may be seen in some myopathies in which the nerves are healthy but the muscle is inexcitable. If no response to either stimulus is

observed, check the equipment and attempt the bipolar method, using two small electrodes to confine the current to the muscle being tested, before making a final statement of "no response to either stimulus."

2. Test results may appear to be normal in the presence of paralysis in the following situations:
   a. Upper motor neuron lesions.
   b. Hysterical paralysis.

Strength–Duration Curve

DESCRIPTION

The strength–duration (SD) curve shows the relationship between the amplitude of a stimulus and the amount of time for which it must be applied to achieve a response. This test is also historical in light of the more sophisticated tests presently available. Like the RD test, it is included here to aid in understanding differences in nerve and muscle responses to different stimuli. The test is performed with mechanically interrupted direct current with stimulus durations varying from 0.05 to 500 msec.

Two quantitative features of the curve that can aid in evaluation and subsequent treatment planning are rheobase and chronaxy. Rheobase is defined as the least amount of current necessary to elicit a minimal visible contraction using an abrupt stimulus of infinite duration. The normal range is 2 to 8 milliamperes (mA). Chronaxy is defined as the minimum time required for an abrupt stimulus of twice rheobase amplitude to elicit a minimal visible contraction. For normally innervated muscle, chronaxy is about 100 μsec. It may be 10 to 100 msec with denervation.

PURPOSE

As an evaluative tool, the SD curve can show the integrity of the nerve muscle complex and the approximate degree of denervation or reinnervation. For planning interventions, establishing chronaxy is valuable in selecting a stimulus appropriate for an individual patient.

ADVANTAGE

The SD curve is a quantitative test and is reproducible.[1]

DISADVANTAGES

1. The test requires special equipment.
2. The test gives information about only those muscle fibers on which the electrode rests and may not give an accurate picture of the total muscle.

INDICATION

The test provides information about the condition of the nerve muscle complex following peripheral neuropathy.

CONTRAINDICATIONS AND PRECAUTIONS

Because this test uses electrical stimulation, the contraindications and precautions are the same as those listed for other modes of electrical stimulation.

INSTRUCTIONS

1. Instruct the patient about what to expect and what you expect of him.
2. Check the skin for sensation and integrity.
3. Position and drape the patient appropriately. The test muscle must be easily visualized and accessible.
4. The examiner should be seated if possible and have all equipment arranged for easy access.
5. Set up a unit designed to perform SD curve testing. Select a stimulus of 100-msec duration, and allow about 0.50 second between stimuli. Be familiar with the other controls on the unit such as scale multipliers and selector switches. Use a foot switch if possible. (These instructions assume the presence of a foot switch. If one is not available, follow the instructions accompanying the equipment.)
6. Turn the power on and allow any necessary warm-up time.
7. Prepare and attach a dispersive electrode to an appropriate area (see general instructions for using electrical stimulators). Make the dispersive electrode positive and the active electrode negative.
8. Prepare an electrode handle with a small button electrode covered with clean gauze and soaked in water. Attach this active electrode to the generator.
9. Initiate the current flow by depressing the foot switch.
10. Locate the motor point of the muscle to be tested. Motor point location involves placing the electrode over the site of the motor point and increasing the current amplitude until a moderate contraction is noted. Release the foot switch to break the circuit, move the electrode to an adjacent area, and examine the size of the contraction there. Continue to search the area until the largest contraction is found without increasing the amplitude. Once the motor point is found, do not move the active electrode throughout the test. Even rolling the active electrode slightly results in testing different muscle fibers and could change the results of the test.
11. Obtain a minimal visible contraction, release the foot switch, and record the stimulus duration and milliammeter reading on a chart similar to the one provided in Figure 15–2.
12. Decrease the stimulus duration by intervals. Depress the foot switch, and readjust the amplitude to maintain the same minimal visible contraction. Continue to record the milliammeter reading for each new duration.

Patient:		Examiner:
Age: Sex:		Interpulse interval:
Date:		

Pulse Duration (milliseconds)	Muscle: Current (mA):	Muscle: Current (mA):
100		
70		
50		
30		
10		
7		
5		
3		
2		
1		
0.8		
0.6		
0.4		
0.3		
0.1		
0.05		

Figure 15–2. Recording form for strength–duration curve testing.

Change the scale multiplier if more current than the scale maximum is required. Remember to multiply the meter reading by the appropriate factor. Do not try to exceed the maximum output of the machine.

13. Check the patient's skin condition and general physiologic responses.
14. Plot the amplitudes on the ordinate and the stimulus durations on the abscissa of the graph in Figure 15–3. Connect the points to form a curve.
15. Determine the rheobase and chronaxy from the graph.
16. Document the durations and amplitudes used, the rheobase and chronaxy, and the patient response.

RESPONSES TO TESTING AND THEIR INTERPRETATION

The shape of the curve is of evaluative and prognostic importance. The curve for normal muscle (Figure 15–4) has a flat right side, showing a consistent threshold to long-duration stimuli. At the left side, as the stimuli become very short, the amplitude required to elicit a response increases sharply.

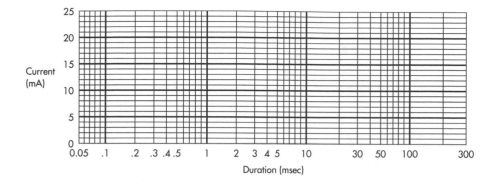

Figure 15–3. Graph to plot strength–duration curve using data from Figure 15–2. (Used with permission of Oxford Instruments; Teca is a trademark of Oxford Instruments.)

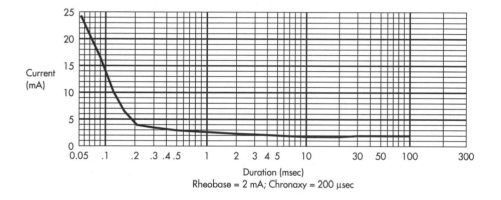

Rheobase = 2 mA; Chronaxy = 200 μsec

Figure 15–4. Strength–duration curve for normal muscle. (Used with permission of Oxford Instruments; Teca is a trademark of Oxford Instruments.)

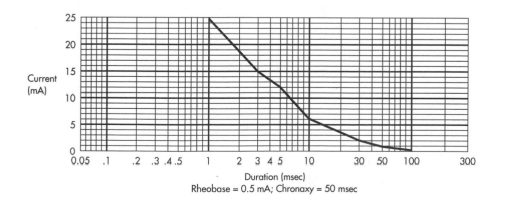
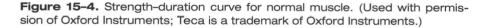

Rheobase = 0.5 mA; Chronaxy = 50 msec

Figure 15–5. Strength–duration curve for denervated muscle. (Used with permission of Oxford Instruments; Teca is a trademark of Oxford Instruments.)

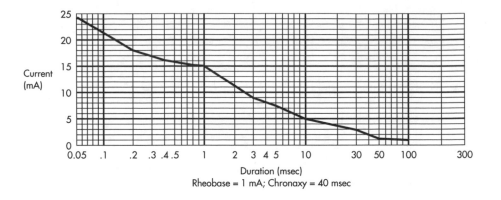
Rheobase = 1 mA; Chronaxy = 40 msec

Figure 15–6. Strength–duration curve for partially denervated muscle. (Used with permission of Oxford Instruments; Teca is a trademark of Oxford Instruments.)

The curve for denervated muscle (Figure 15–5) is "shifted to the right," indicating the loss of ability to respond to short-duration stimuli. It is markedly sloped, indicating that an increase in amplitude is needed each time the duration is shortened. Chronaxy is longer, and the rheobase may initially be lower.

The curve for partially denervated muscle (Figure 15–6) displays a combination of the features of the curves for both normal and denervated muscle. Response to shorter duration stimuli is present, but chronaxy may still be lengthened. A kink in the curve is the first sign of reinnervation, followed by widening of the curve, and finally shifting back to the left and smoothing.

Nerve Conduction Velocity Testing

DESCRIPTION

There are many aspects of nerve conduction velocity (NCV) testing, including motor nerve conduction velocity (MNCV), sensory nerve conduction velocity (SNCV), F waves, H reflexes, and somatosensory evoked potentials. The purpose of this discussion is to provide a fundamental understanding of MNCV and SNCV. For other aspects of NCV, which are beyond the scope of this book, refer to more comprehensive texts.[2,3]

MNCV testing is a measure of the speed of conduction of a nerve impulse along the course of a peripheral nerve. The procedure uses an electromyograph that is equipped with an amplifier, computer, monitor, and stimulator. The test may be performed on any nerve that is superficial at least twice in its course and has a distally located reference muscle that is innervated exclusively by the nerve of interest. The test is designed to eliminate the time delay at the neuromuscular junction. Therefore, the nerve is stimulated in two places, and the time for each stimulus to reach the reference muscle is measured. Then the speed between the two stimulation sites is calculated.

Sensory conduction times can be measured in either an antidromic or orthodromic manner on superficial peripheral sensory nerves. In either motor or sensory conduction velocity measurements, only the velocity of the fastest conducting fibers are actually measured.

PURPOSE

Nerve conduction velocity testing is used to detect the condition of the nerve. It is particularly useful in compression lesions of the peripheral nerves. Sensory velocities are highly sensitive measures of early peripheral neuropathy, identifying changes in velocity that occur early in the progression of the condition.

CONTRAINDICATIONS

Because the test involves electrical stimulation, please refer to the contraindications listed for other modes of electrical stimulation.

INSTRUCTIONS

Motor Nerve Conduction Velocity

1. Instruct the patient regarding what to expect and what you expect of her.
2. Check the patient's skin for sensation and integrity.
3. Perform the test on both involved and uninvolved sides. Begin with the uninvolved side.
4. Position and drape the patient for comfort and modesty. Be sure that the extremity is positioned so that the nerve is at its true length and all stimulation sites are accessible. For example, to test the ulnar nerve, the patient should be positioned supine with the shoulder in about 90° of abduction and the elbow flexed to 90° of flexion. This position takes the slack out of the nerve and more closely approximates its true length.[2]
5. Determine the sites for stimulation, the reference muscle, and the site for the ground electrode. The ground electrode helps reject noise signals and is usually placed on a bony prominence between the stimulating and recording electrodes (Figure 15–7).
6. Prepare all electrode sites by abrading them and cleansing the skin with alcohol to decrease the skin impedance.
7. Prepare the recording and ground electrodes with conductive paste or gel and fasten them to the skin firmly with adhesive tape. The recording electrode should be placed with the cathode over the belly of the reference muscle and the anode distal to it over the tendon of insertion. Attach both recording and ground electrodes to the preamplifier.
8. Prepare an electromyograph that allows a frequency response of 10 to 10,000 Hz. Set the gain for 1000 to 5000 microvolts per division (start with 2000 µV/div) and the sweep for 2 to 5 msec per division.[4] Set the stimulator to produce a direct current stimulus of 0.1 msec at a rate of 1 per second.
9. Attach the lead wires of the stimulator to the appropriate terminals of the electromyograph. Prepare the stimulator electrodes with conductive

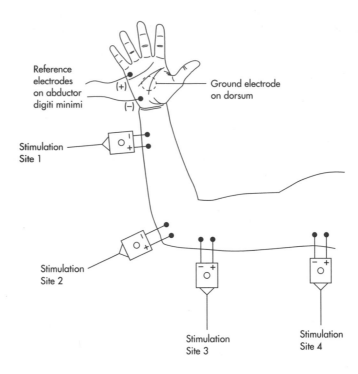

Figure 15–7. Stimulation and pick-up electrode sites for motor nerve conduction velocity testing of the ulnar nerve.

paste on the tips. Firmly place the stimulator along the course of the nerve where it is superficial with the cathode placed distally and the anode placed proximally.

10. Increase the current amplitude until the evoked response in the reference muscle is maximal.

11. On the computer monitor, a stimulus artifact appears at the moment of stimulation. Mark the onset of the evoked compound action potential, and measure the latency from the stimulus artifact to the onset of the response (Figure 15–8). Record the time in milliseconds as Latency 1, and mark the site of the stimulating cathode with a skin pencil.

12. Repeat steps 9 through 11 at a more proximal site along the nerve. Record this latency as Latency 2, and mark the second stimulation site. Be sure that the size and shape of the evoked potential is consistent at each stimulation site.

13. Remove the equipment, and check the patient's skin for integrity.

14. To calculate the conduction velocity, measure the distance in millimeters between the two stimulation cathode sites. Divide the distance by the difference in milliseconds between the two latencies.

$$\frac{\text{Distance between stimulation sites (mm)}}{\text{Latency 2} - \text{Latency 1 (msec)}} = \text{velocity in m/sec}$$

15. Clean the gel and marks from the patient's skin.

16. Repeat the test on the contralateral side.

17. Document the potential diagnosis, the nerve tested, distal latencies, NCV for each segment calculated, peak-to-peak amplitude of the evoked response, and any other patient response.

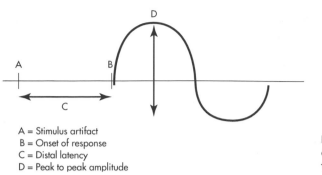

A = Stimulus artifact
B = Onset of response
C = Distal latency
D = Peak to peak amplitude

Figure 15-8. Evoked compound action potential.

Sensory Nerve Conduction Velocity

1. Prepare the patient, skin, and electrodes in the same way as for motor conduction measurements.

2. For orthodromic sensory conduction measurement, place the stimulating electrodes distally in the distribution. For example, to test the sensory conduction of the ulnar nerve, the electrodes are ring electrodes placed on the little finger. Place the negative stimulating electrode proximal to the positive stimulating electrode. Place the recording electrodes proximally, along the course of the nerve with the recording cathode placed distally to the recording anode (Figure 15–9). For antidromic conduction measurements, stimulate along the course of the nerve, cathode distally, and record the response with the ring electrodes that are placed on the little finger, cathode proximally. The ground electrode is located as for motor velocity testing.

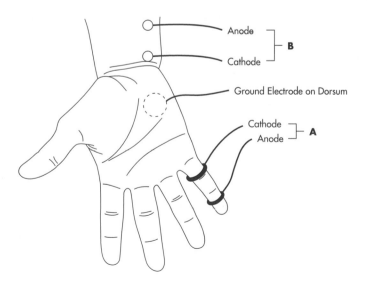

Figure 15-9. Electrode placement sites for sensory nerve conduction velocity of the ulnar nerve. For orthodromic testing, the ring electrodes (A) are the stimulating electrodes, with the pick-up proximally along the nerve (B). For antidromic testing, stimulation is performed along the nerve (B), and the response is recorded with the ring electrodes (A).

3. Prepare the electromyograph to produce the same stimulus as for motor conduction. Set the gain for 5 to 20 microvolts per division and the sweep speed for 1 to 2 milliseconds per division.[4]
4. Turn the current amplitude only high enough to produce a sensory stimulus.
5. Measure the latency on the computer monitor from the stimulus artifact to the *peak* of the single phase of the evoked response. Because there is no junctional delay for sensory testing, sensory latencies may be used to compute a velocity or may be used alone.
6. Remove the apparatus, and clean the patient's skin.
7. Document the patient's potential diagnosis, the nerve tested, distal latencies, NCV for each segment calculated, peak-to-peak amplitude of the evoked response, and any other patient response.

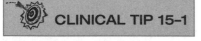

CLINICAL TIP 15-1

Electrode Placement for Electrophysiologic Evaluation

To give meaning to comparison of results, especially distal latencies, standardize the distance between stimulating and reference electrodes.

RESPONSES TO TESTING AND THEIR INTERPRETATION

All results of conduction velocity testing should be compared with the patient's intact extremity, previous test results, or normal values established for the laboratory in which the test was performed. Velocities are slower for very young or very old patients and if the temperature of the room is cold. Normal upper extremity motor velocities are usually 45 to 65 m/sec, and lower extremity velocities are slightly slower.

1. Nerve conduction may be absent, indicating a complete failure of conduction along the course of the nerve between the stimulating and recording electrodes.
2. Conduction velocities can be slowed along the entire nerve, indicating a demyelinating condition such as Gullain-Barré syndrome.
3. Conduction velocities may be slowed along a segment of the nerve, indicating a local pathology such as compression. Velocities in more distal segments may be normal.
4. In conditions involving degeneration of some axons but not others, conduction velocities may remain normal, but the evoked responses are diminished.
5. Patients with paralysis from upper motor neuron causes or hysteria have normal nerve conduction velocities.

REFERENCES

1. Nelson RM, Hunt GC. Strength–duration curve: intrarater and inter-rater reliability. *Phys Ther.* 1981;61:894–897.
2. Echternach JL. *Introduction to Electromyography and Nerve Conduction Testing: A Laboratory Manual.* Thorofare, NJ: Slack Incorporated; 1994.
3. Goodgold J, Eberstein A. *Electrodiagnosis of Neuromuscular Disease.* Baltimore: Williams & Wilkins; 1983.
4. Nelson RM, Nestor DE. Electrophysiological evaluation: an overview. In: Nelson RM, Currier DP, eds. *Clinical Electrotherapy.* 2nd ed. Norwalk, CT: Appleton & Lange; 1991: 331–383.

ADDITIONAL READINGS

Arieff AJ. Newer concepts of electrodiagnosis in peripheral nerve injuries. *Arch Phys Med Rehabil.* 1948;29:571–578.

Aulick LH. The galvanic tetanus ratio test. *Phys Ther.* 1967;47:933–936.

Bhala R. Electrodiagnosis of ulnar nerve lesions at the elbow. *Arch Phys Med Rehabil.* 1976; 57:206–212.

Bouman HD, Shaffer KJ. Physiological basis of electrical stimulation of human muscle and its clinical application. *Phys Ther Rev.* 1957;37:207–223.

Campbell JM. Electrodiagnostics revisited: a powerful evaluation tool. *Top Acute Care Trauma Rehabil.* 1988;3:10–26.

Currier DP. Placement of recording electrode in median and peroneal nerve conduction studies. *Phys Ther.* 1975;55:365–370.

Echternach JL. The use of conduction velocity measurements as an evaluative tool. In: Wolf SL, ed. *Electrotherapy.* New York: Churchill Livingstone; 1981:73–97.

Echternach JL, Sidel L. Progressive current testing in peripheral nerve injuries and nerve root compression. *Phys Ther.* 1968;48:1383–1391.

Hamilton GF, Harrison E. A paint-on silver electrode and its application to electrodiagnosis. *Phys Ther.* 1969;49:1382–1384.

Harding C, Halar E. Motor and sensory ulnar nerve conduction velocities: effect of elbow position. *Arch Phys Med Rehabil.* 1983;64:227–232.

Humphries R, Currier DP. Variables in recording motor conduction of the radial nerve. *Phys Ther.* 1976;56:809–813.

Kellogg R. Electrophysiologic evaluation. *Clin Manage.* 1991;11(4):34–42.

Lucci R. The effects of age on motor-nerve conduction velocity. *Phys Ther.* 1969;49: 973–976.

Mitz M, Gokulananda T, DiBenedetto M, Klingbeil G. Median nerve determinations: analysis of two techniques. *Arch Phys Med Rehabil.* 1984;65:191–193.

Electromyographic Biofeedback

Wendy Jensen Poe and Antoinette P. Sander

DESCRIPTION

Biofeedback is the use of instrumentation to provide objective information (feedback) to an individual about a physiologic function or response so that a person can become aware of the response. Electromyographic (EMG) biofeedback is based on the principles of electromyography, which monitors motor unit action potentials (MUAPs) during muscle contraction. Biofeedback devices measure the amplitude of MUAPs in microvolts (μV). The biofeedback unit amplifies, filters, rectifies, integrates, and displays the MUAPs in audio and visual formats. The magnitude of the contraction reflects the number of motor units firing, the electrode size and placement, and the distance of the active fibers from the recording electrodes.[1]

Two parameters are adjusted in EMG biofeedback treatment: the gain/sensitivity and the threshold/goal. Biofeedback equipment displays the output voltage in a variety of ways: an oscilloscope screen, a bar graph, a liquid crystal display (LCD), a number graph, and so on. The gain is the amplification of the signal to a size that may be displayed. High gain settings are more sensitive, are scaled as low microvoltages, and are used to display minimal MUAPs. Low gain settings are less sensitive, are scaled as high microvoltages, and are used to display many MUAPs. Adjusting the gain/sensitivity allows the signal to be viewed in the middle of the display screen (Figure 16–1). Simple equipment may offer only high and low gain settings; more sophisticated equipment may offer multiple gain settings.

The threshold/goal is the predetermined level of muscle activity at which audio and/or visual feedback is given. This provides a clear goal for the patient and is altered by the practitioner to achieve motor recruitment or inhibition. Visual feedback may be sophisticated computer graphics or a simple LCD. Auditory feedback may be a click or a tone that sounds when threshold is reached or that becomes quiet when threshold is reached.

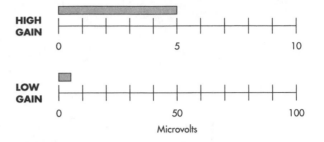

Figure 16–1. Output display. Two scales for setting gain/sensitivity are diagrammed with a 5-μV signal shown on both scales. In this example, the high gain scale more accurately displays the 5-μV reading.

Biofeedback units come with a range of enhancements. Many EMG biofeedback units have multichannel capabilities so that agonist, antagonist, and synergistic muscles can be monitored simultaneously, allowing both recruitment and inhibition feedback during larger scale functional movement patterns. Some instrumentation is available to monitor EMG output under water. In addition, EMG and neuromuscular stimulation can be combined in some units. The threshold is set for recruitment. When the threshold is achieved, neuromuscular stimulation is activated for an additional strengthening contraction.

PURPOSE AND EFFECTS

EMG biofeedback changes MUAPs into auditory and/or visual cues for the purpose of *increasing* or *decreasing* voluntary activity. Biofeedback is a tool to enhance motor learning by providing feedback about performance until motor skills develop sufficiently so that no external feedback is required.[2] By making use of the auditory and visual feedback about the electrical activity produced by the muscles, a patient is able to monitor physiologic events and learn to recognize desired responses, a form of operant conditioning. Biofeedback provides positive reinforcement for motor learning by rewarding small changes in motor behavior. It is an objective, continuous, timely response to the patient's efforts to control muscle output. Feedback can be given without the constant presence of the practitioner, which makes it cost effective.

For EMG biofeedback to be effective, the patient using the equipment should be mentally alert with thought processes generally intact, have the ability to produce voluntary contraction of the muscle being monitored, and be motivated to work with the equipment.

INDICATIONS

1. Motor recruitment: conditions in which the goal is to increase the EMG signal from the targeted muscle(s).
   a. Paresis resulting from lower motor neuron pathology (e.g., recovering from peripheral nerve injuries, Bell's palsy,[3] Guillain-Barré[4]).

b. Paresis resulting from upper motor neuron lesions (e.g., incomplete spinal cord lesions,[5] hemiparesis secondary to cerebrovascular accident,[6] traumatic brain injury, cerebral palsy).

c. Specificity training or strengthening in a variety of orthopedic cases (e.g., vastus medialis oblique [VMO] recruitment, scapular stabilization training, rotator cuff repair, tendon transfers[7,8]).

d. Hysterical paralysis.

e. Perineal muscle reeducation as treatment for urinary incontinence.[9–11]

2. Motor inhibition: conditions in which the goal is to decrease the EMG signal from the targeted muscle(s).

a. Inhibition of spastic or hypertonic muscles that are interfering with recruitment of the primary agonist of a functional movement or movement pattern. Simultaneous recruitment of antagonistic muscles with agonist inhibition is recommended in upper motor neuron pathology[12,13] (e.g., cerebrovascular accident or other upper motor neuron pathology, cerebral palsy,[14] spinal cord injury, traumatic brain injury).

b. Inhibition of tight muscles that are interfering with the functional range of motion of a joint.

c. Inhibition of muscle dystonia (e.g., torticollis,[15] reflex sympathetic dystrophy–related dystonia).

d. Reduction of faulty compensatory or substitution recruitment patterns during specificity training in a variety of orthopedic cases (e.g., vastus lateralis inhibition during VMO reeducation, upper trapezius inhibition during shoulder rehabilitation or postural reeducation, abdominal-gluteal inhibition during urinary incontinence and pelvic floor retraining).

3. Total body relaxation: conditions of generalized pain or stress in which the goal is to decrease undesirable muscle tension and achieve relaxation and stress reduction.

a. Pain control (e.g., headache,[16,17] musculoskeletal pain,[18] temporomandibular joint syndrome,[19] back pain[20]).

b. Stress management (e.g., anxiety[21,22]).

PRECAUTIONS

There are no specific contraindications to the use of EMG biofeedback. Skin irritation can occur from the sensor or electrode gel or tape with prolonged use.

INSTRUCTIONS

Before beginning any treatment, become familiar with the EMG biofeedback instrument controls for gain/sensitivity, threshold/goal, and audio-visual functions. Self-treatment ensures understanding of the equipment.

General Procedures

1. Select the appropriate muscle or muscle group to monitor depending on the desired goal.

2. Most current EMG biofeedback instruments are designed to be used with disposable, pregelled adhesive electrodes. When using reusable electrodes, make sure the electrodes are clean and free of conductive gel residue before applying fresh gel and adhering with tape.

3. Prepare the skin by cleaning with alcohol or lightly abrading the electrode sites using gauze, fine-grade sandpaper, or conducting spray.

4. Select the appropriate electrode size. Electrodes are sometimes referred to as sensors because they detect muscle activity rather than introduce a stimulus. There are two active electrodes and a ground. Small electrodes (1 cm) pick up over a smaller area and have greater specificity, but they also have more skin impedance. Large electrodes (>1 cm) pick up over a larger area and have less specificity, and they also have less skin impedance.

5. Determine the appropriate electrode placement. Place active or signal electrodes over the motor point of the muscle being monitored and parallel to the muscle fibers. Be aware that the skin may move over the muscle during contraction and alter the territory being monitored. Placement over adipose tissue may attenuate the signal. Place the ground electrode over a bony prominence or noncontractile tissue, if available. Electrode and ground electrode placement should remain consistent across treatment sessions.

6. Select the appropriate electrode spacing. Close spacing (1 to 2 cm) monitors fewer MUAPs, provides more specificity, and limits cross-talk from adjacent or antagonist muscles. Wide spacing (2 to 5 cm) monitors more MUAPs, gives broader EMG responses, and increases the possibility of cross-talk from surrounding muscles. Use a spacing that optimizes the signal and minimizes the cross-talk.[23]

7. Wrapping the electrodes and connecting wires securely with an elastic bandage may reduce the movement artifact.

Motor Recruitment

Goal: To provide feedback to increase desirable motor unit activity, thus increasing voluntary motor control.

Procedure:

1. Keeping the goal of the session in mind, position the patient comfortably to receive the audio-visual feedback.

2. Explain the procedure to the patient.

3. Prepare and apply the two signal electrodes securely to the muscle to be recruited. Apply the ground to a convenient site.

4. Adjust the initial gain/sensitivity at a level that registers the available active muscle contraction in the middle of the scale. This initial microvolt reading is the "baseline" of this treatment session. One goal in recruitment is to increase this baseline from session to session.

5. Determine whether audio and/or visual feedback will be given, and adjust the machine to provide the appropriate feedback.

6. Set the initial threshold/goal just above the "baseline" level of voluntary motor response. The patient must then work to increase the motor output to reach the threshold/goal and receive the audio-visual feedback. Adjust the threshold to a level that challenges the patient but still allows success to provide positive reinforcement for motor learning.

⊙ CLINICAL TIP 16–1

Tips to Optimize Treatment With Electromyographic Biofeedback

- Decrease skin impedance prior to electrode application.
- Place the recording electrodes parallel to the muscle fibers.
- Threshold is the predetermined level of muscle activity at which feedback is given.
- For muscle recruitment, decrease the gain as the muscle gets stronger.
- For muscle inhibition, increase the gain as the muscle relaxes.
- Keep electrode placement consistent from session to session.
- If electrodes are to be reused, replace them on their plastic coated paper and store them in a sealed bag.

7. Instruct the patient to contract the target muscle(s) using facilitation techniques as appropriate (e.g., tapping, vibration, weightbearing, cross facilitation, mass patterns, overflow, quick stretch, etc.).
8. Shape the threshold/goal by moving to higher numbers within the gain scale.
9. Shape the gain by decreasing the sensitivity range of the EMG unit to higher numbers as the patient is able to recruit more MUAPs. This "shaping" procedure allows training to start with minimal response and to make the criteria for success gradually more difficult until the desired goals are attained.
10. As motor recruitment increases and short-term goals are met, begin to incorporate functional movement patterns into treatment.
11. Continue EMG monitoring to achieve the desired goals, gradually weaning from the external feedback to internal feedback.
12. Remove the electrodes from the patient, and clean any adhesive residue from the skin. Perform any indicated posttreatment reassessment procedures.
13. Document electrode placement and spacing, progress in gain/sensitivity and threshold settings, microvolt recruitment levels, spontaneous recruitment, sustained recruitment, positioning toward function, duration of treatment, and so on.

Dosage

Treatment session length depends on patient participation, patient fatigue, and outcomes achieved. In general, work with the patient for 15 to 45 minutes. The frequency and duration are dependent on progress toward short-term and long-term functional goals. Discontinue biofeedback when the patient can perform the desired motor pattern.

Home Use

Instruct the patient in a specific out-of-therapy exercise to reinforce the motor recruitment process. Portable EMG units, which are available for home use, may be considered in some cases.

Motor Inhibition

Goal: Provide feedback to decrease undesirable motor unit activity that may be interfering with functional movement.
Procedure:

1. Keeping the goal of the session in mind, position the patient comfortably to receive the audio-visual feedback.
2. Explain procedures to the patient.
3. Prepare and apply two signal electrodes securely to the muscle to be inhibited or relaxed. Apply the ground to a nearby bony prominence.
4. Adjust the initial gain/sensitivity setting to the level that registers the current resting muscle activity in the center of the scale. This initial microvolt reading is the "baseline" of this treatment session. One goal in inhibition is to decrease this baseline from session to session.
5. Determine whether audio and/or visual feedback will be given, and adjust the machine to provide the appropriate feedback.

6. Set the initial threshold/goal just below the "baseline" level of perceived relaxed or resting motor response. Determine a level that challenges the patient but still allows for success to provide positive reinforcement for motor learning. By doing this, the patient must maintain the relaxation or further relax the target muscle to receive positive feedback.

7. Instruct the patient to relax the target area using inhibition or relaxation techniques as appropriate.

8. Shape the threshold/goal by moving to lower microvolt settings within the gain scale as the patient is able to relax the target muscle.

9. Shape the gain by increasing the sensitivity range of the EMG unit to lower numbers as the patient is able to relax the target muscle further.

10. As target muscle MUAPs are diminished and goals are attained, move to more functionally challenging positions and dynamic activities. Continue EMG monitoring to achieve desired goals, gradually weaning from external feedback to internal feedback.

11. Remove electrodes, and clean any adhesive residue from the skin. Perform any indicated posttreatment reassessment procedures.

12. Document electrode placement and spacing, progress in gain/sensitivity and threshold settings, microvolt inhibition levels, positioning toward function, treatment duration, and so on.

Dosage

Treatment session length is 15 to 45 minutes, depending on patient participation, patient fatigue, and outcomes achieved. Frequency and duration depend on progress toward short-term and long-term functional goals.

Home Use

Instruct the patient in a specific out-of-therapy exercise to reinforce the motor inhibition process. Consider teaching the patient to use a portable biofeedback unit when not in the clinic.

Total Body Relaxation

Goal: To train the patient in recognizing the sensations of total body relaxation.
Procedure:

1. Position the patient to receive the visual-auditory feedback comfortably and as relaxed as possible in a *quiet* area.

2. Explain procedures to the patient.

3. Prepare and apply the two signal electrodes securely to the muscle to be monitored. Apply the ground to a convenient site. There are three muscles or groups of muscles chosen for total body relaxation biofeedback:
   a. Forearm extensors.
   b. Frontalis muscle.
   c. Specific muscle groups that are tense (e.g., trapezius, paraspinals, masseter).

4. Instruct the patient to relax as much as possible for 5 minutes without any audio-visual feedback. Adjust the initial gain/sensitivity setting to the level that registers the current resting muscle activity in the center of the scale. This initial microvolt reading is the "baseline" of this treat-

ment session. One goal in total body relaxation is to decrease this baseline from session to session.

5. Determine whether audio and/or visual feedback will be given and adjust the machine to provide the appropriate feedback.

6. Set the initial threshold/goal below the baseline level of perceived relaxed or resting motor response at a level that challenges the patient but still allows for success. By doing this, the patient must maintain the relaxation or further relax the target muscle to receive positive feedback.

7. Instruct the patient to relax as much as possible. Relaxation techniques and diaphragmatic breathing may be incorporated into the biofeedback session. Suggested relaxation techniques include progressive relaxation, meditation, autogenic phrases, and visualization. A script for one of the more common general relaxation techniques is included at the end of this chapter.[24]

8. Shape the threshold/goal by moving to lower microvolt settings within the gain scale as the patient is able to achieve deeper levels of relaxation.

9. Shape the gain by increasing the sensitivity range of the EMG unit to lower numbers as the patient is able to relax further.

10. Microvolt goals for total body relaxation range from 1 to 3.5 μV.[25]

11. As relaxation is achieved, progress the treatment by:
    a. Introducing mental stressors during the training sessions.
    b. Relaxing without feedback.
    c. Relaxing quickly and frequently in daily life.

12. Remove electrodes, and clean any adhesive residue from the skin. Perform any indicated posttreatment reassessment procedures.

13. Document electrode placement and spacing, progress in gain/sensitivity and threshold settings, microvolt relaxation levels, treatment duration, progress toward stress management, and so on.

Dosage

Treatment session length depends on patient participation, patient fatigue, and outcomes achieved. Plan to work with the patient from 30 to 60 minutes. Frequency and duration depend on progress toward short-term and long-term functional goals.

Home Use

Home practice of relaxation skills greatly enhances the biofeedback sessions.

RESPONSES TO TREATMENT

Whole body relaxation decreases sympathetic nervous system activity, potentially lowering heart rate, blood pressure, and respiratory rate. A state of deep relaxation usually brings a feeling of well being accompanied by an awareness of muscle tension and muscle relaxation and a release of anxiety. Deep relaxation in highly anxious or depressed clients can result in emotional lability.

Patients with diabetes need to monitor blood glucose levels when practicing deep relaxation techniques.[26] Increased sympathetic activity that accompanies stress tends to decrease the body's secretion of insulin, resulting in an increase in blood glucose levels. Conversely, deep relaxation may result in an increased secretion of insulin and a subsequent decrease in blood glucose levels.

SCRIPT FOR PROGRESSIVE NEUROMUSCULAR RELAXATION

Read the following script slowly, taking 20 to 30 minutes to guide the patient in progressive relaxation.

The goal of this technique is to achieve overall relaxation by releasing muscle tension throughout the body. To appreciate the difference between muscle tension and muscle relaxation, you will be asked to contract specific muscle groups and then to release the tension. This contraction-relaxation may be repeated two to three times. The focus is always on how the muscle and the body feel during the relaxation.

1. Begin with several slow, deep breaths, letting your abdomen rise as you breathe in and fall as you breathe out.
2. Now focus your attention on your shoulders. Shrug both shoulders as high as you can, and feel the tension created across the top of your shoulders.
3. Let go, release the tension, and let your shoulders drop down. Notice the difference between the feelings of tension and the feelings of relaxation.
4. Shrug your shoulders half way up this time. Where is the tension created? Let go of the tension, dropping your shoulders down.
5. Now imagine you are lifting your shoulders without moving. Feel the tension created and let it go.
6. Find any remaining tension across the top of your shoulders, and release that tension. Focus all your attention on the feelings associated with relaxation flowing into these muscles.
7. Squeeze your shoulder blades together, and notice the tension created across your back.
8. Let go and release the tension.
9. Squeeze your shoulder blades together again, but only half as hard as before. Let go, releasing the tension and focusing on the feelings of relaxation.
10. Now focus on any remaining tension across your shoulder blades. Let go of this tightness, letting the shoulders feel more and more relaxed.
11. Make a fist, and tighten your right hand and arm as much as you can. Feel the tension, and then let it go.
12. Tighten your right hand and arm again, but only half as tight as before. Let the tension go, and focus on the difference between the feelings of tension and feelings of relaxation.
13. Let go of any remaining tension in your right hand, arm, and shoulder.
14. Notice any difference in the feelings of tension in the right arm and the left arm.
15. Make a fist, and tighten your left hand and arm as much as you can. Feel the tension, and then let it go.
16. Tighten your left hand and arm again, but only half as tight as before. Let the tension go, and focus on the difference between the feelings of tension and feelings of relaxation.
17. Let go of any remaining tension in your left hand, arm, and shoulder.
18. Take several slow, deep breaths, letting your abdomen rise as you breathe in and fall as you breathe out.

19. Feel your arms and shoulders become more and more relaxed.
20. Focus your attention on your face.
21. Wrinkle your forehead by raising your eyebrows up. Feel the tension and release it.
22. Wrinkle your forehead again, making half the tension you did before. Release the tension, feeling your forehead become relaxed and smooth.
23. Find and release any remaining tension in your forehead.
24. Close your eyes tightly and feel the tension around your eyes. Release the tension.
25. Close your eyes again, half as tight as before. Release this tension and focus on the difference between tension and relaxation.
26. Clench your jaw by biting your teeth together and notice the area of tension in your jaw.
27. Release this tension, let your teeth come apart in the back and rest your tongue on the roof of your mouth. In this position, release any remaining tension across your jaw.
28. Take several slow, deep breaths, letting your abdomen rise as you breathe in and fall as you breathe out. Feel the muscles of your face become smooth and more and more relaxed.
29. Focus your attention on your lower back and legs.
30. Squeeze your buttocks together tightly and feel tension in your hips and low back. Release the tension.
31. Squeeze your buttocks together again, but not as tight as before. Feel the tension, and then release it. Notice the difference between the feelings of tension and the feelings of relaxation.
32. Find any remaining tension in your buttocks and lower back, and release the tension.
33. Tighten the muscles in your right leg by straightening your knee. Feel the tension, and then release it.
34. Tighten the muscles in your right leg again, but half as much as before. Release the tension.
35. Feel any remaining tension in the right leg and release the tension.
36. Focus on the feelings of relaxation in the right leg.
37. Notice any difference in feelings of relaxation in the right leg and the left leg.
38. Tighten the muscles in your left leg by straightening your knee. Feel the tension, and then release it.
39. Tighten the muscles in your left leg again, but half as much as before. Release the tension.
40. Feel any remaining tension in the left leg and release the tension.
41. Focus on the feelings of relaxation in the left leg.
42. Take several deep, slow breaths. Scan your body from the top of your head to the tips of your toes. With each exhaled breath, release any remaining tension you may find, letting relaxation flow throughout your body. Notice the position of your muscles when they are relaxed, and the sensations in your body as relaxation takes place. As you learn the relaxed position of your muscles, you will begin to function throughout your day with less tension. Savor your relaxed feeling for a few minutes. Breathe easily and regularly. When you are ready, slowly open your eyes and become aware of your surroundings. Stretch and resume your activities.

REFERENCES

1. Binder-Macleod SA. Electromyographic biofeedback to improve voluntary motor control. In: Robinson AJ, Snyder-Mackler L. *Clinical Electrophysiology.* Baltimore: Williams & Wilkins. 1995:435–449.

2. Krebs DE, Behr DW. Biofeedback. In: O'Sullivan SB, Schmitz TJ. *Physical Rehabilitation: Assessment and Treatment.* Philadelphia: F.A. Davis. 1994:707–724.

3. Ross B, Nedzelski JM, McLean JA. Efficacy of feedback training in long-standing facial nerve paresis. *Laryngoscope.* 1991;101:744–750.

4. Ince LP, Brenes J, Carmen C. EMG biofeedback to patients with Guillain-Barré syndrome. *Rehabil Psychol.* 1987;32:155–163.

5. Brucker BS, Bulaeva NV. Biofeedback effect on electromyography responses in patients with spinal cord injury. *Arch Phys Med Rehabil.* 1996;77:133–137.

6. Intiso D, Santilli V, Grasso MG, et al. Rehabilitation of walking with electromyographic biofeedback in foot-drop after stroke. *Stroke.* 1994;25:1186–1192.

7. Headley BJ. Chronic pain management. In: O'Sullivan SB, Schmitz. TJ. *Physical Rehabilitation: Assessment and Treatment.* Philadelphia: F.A. Davis; 1994:577–602.

8. Levitt R, Deisinger JA, Remondet WJ, et al. EMG feedback assisted post operative rehabilitation of minor arthroscopic knee surgeries. *J Sports Med Phys Fitness.* 1995;35:218–223.

9. Tries J, Brubaker L. Application of biofeedback in the treatment of urinary incontinence. *Prof Psychol Res Prac.* 1996;27:554–560.

10. Workman DE, Cassisi JE, Dougherty MC. Validation of surface EMG as a measure of intravaginal and intra-abdominal activity: implications for biofeedback-assisted Kegel exercises. *Psychophysiology.* 1993;30:120–125.

11. McIntosh LJ, Frahm JD, Mallett VT, Richardson DA. Pelvic floor rehabilitation in the treatment of incontinence. *J Reprod Med.* 1993;38:662–666.

12. Gowland C, deBruin H, Basmajian JV, et al. Agonist and antagonist activity during voluntary upper-limb movement in patients with stroke. *Phys Ther.* 1992;72:624–633.

13. Wolf SL, Catlin PA, Blanton S, et al. Overcoming limitations in elbow movement in the presence of antagonist hyperactivity. *Phys Ther.* 1994;74:826–835.

14. Colborne GR, Wright FV, Naumann S. Feedback of triceps surae EMG in gait of children with cerebral palsy: a controlled study. *Arch Phys Med Rehabil.* 1994;75:40–45.

15. Jahanshahi M, Sartory G, Marsden CD. EMG biofeedback treatment of torticollis: a controlled outcome study. *Biofeed Self Regul.* 1991;16:413–448.

16. Arena JG, Bruno GM, Hannah SL, Meador KJ. A comparison of frontal electromyographic biofeedback training, trapezius electromyographic biofeedback training, and progressive muscle relaxation therapy in the treatment of tension headache. *Headache.* 1995;35:411–419.

17. Cott A, Parkinson W, Fabich M, et al. Long-term efficacy of combined relaxation: biofeedback treatments for chronic headache. *Pain.* 1992;51:49–56.

18. Flor H, Birbaumer N. Comparison of the efficacy of electromyographic biofeedback, cognitive-behavioral therapy, and conservative medical interventions in the treatment of chronic musculoskeletal pain. *J Consult Clin Psychol.* 1993;61:653–658.

19. Turk DC, Zaki HS, Rudy TE. Effects of intraoral appliance and biofeedback/stress management alone and in combination in treating pain and depression in patients with temporomandibular disorders. *J Prost Dent.* 1993;70:158–164.

20. Shihab S, Parek M. Biofeedback and back muscle strengthening. *Spine.* 1990;15:510–513.

21. Rice KM, Blanchard EB, Purcell M. Biofeedback treatments of generalized anxiety disorder: preliminary results. *Biofeed Self Regul.* 1993;18:93–105.

22. Hurley JD, Meminger SR. A relapse-prevention program: effects of electromyographic training on high and low levels of state and trait anxiety. *Percept Mot Skills.* 1992;74:699–705.

23. Hecox B, Mehreteab TA, Weisberg J. *Physical Agents.* Norwalk, Conn: Appleton & Lange; 1994.

24. Basmajian JV. *Biofeedback Principles and Practice for Clinicians*. Baltimore: Williams & Wilkins; 1989:169–185.
25. Basmajian JV. *Biofeedback Principles and Practice for Clinicians*. Baltimore: Williams & Wilkins; 1989:176.
26. McGrady A, Bailey B. Biofeedback-assisted relaxation and diabetes mellitus. In: Schwartz, MS. *Biofeedback*. New York: Guilford Press; 1996:471–489.

ADDITIONAL READINGS

McNulty WH, Gevirtz RN, Hubbard DR, Berkoff GM. Needle electromyographic evaluation of trigger point response to a psychological stressor. *Psychophysiology.* 1994;31: 313–316.

Moreland J, Thomson MA. Efficacy of electromyographic biofeedback compared with conventional physical therapy for upper extremity function in patients following stroke: a research overview and meta-analysis. *Phys Ther.* 1994;74:534–543.

Newton-John TR, Spence SH, Schotte D. Cognitive-behavioural therapy versus EMG biofeedback in the treatment of chronic low back pain. *Behav Res Ther.* 1995;33:691–697.

Spence SH, Sharpe L, Newton-John T. Champion D. Effect of EMG biofeedback compared to applied relaxation training with chronic, upper extremity cumulative trauma disorders. *Pain.* 1995;63:199–206.

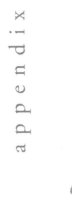

Electromagnetic Spectrum

0.01nm	0.14nm	12nm	180nm	290nm	320nm	400nm		800nm	1500nm	15,000nm	10cm	1m	3m	30m	30,000m

Cosmic Rays	Gamma Rays	X-rays		UVC	UVB	UVA	Violet Indigo Blue Green Yellow Orange Red	Short or Near	Long or Far		Microwave	Radar	Shortwave		Low Frequency Stimulating Currents
					Ultraviolet		Visible Light		Infrared						

One nanometer (nm) = 10^{-9} meter (m)
One hertz = one cycle per second

Laws Governing Dosage of Electromagnetic Radiation

Grotthus Draper Law

Only those waves that are absorbed can cause secondary effects.

Bunsen Roscoe Law of Reciprocity

The intensity and duration of the dose of radiant energy are inversely proportional.

$$E = It$$

where:

E = energy
I = intensity
t = time

To keep the amount of energy constant, an increase in intensity must be accompanied by a decrease in duration and vice versa.

Inverse Square Law

The intensity of the waves from a point source varies inversely with the square of the distance from the source. Thus, if the distance of the irradiated surface from the source is increased, the same amount of energy must cover more area and is relatively weaker.

For example, if the distance from point source A (Figure B–1) is increased from 1 foot to 3 feet, the area irradiated is nine times as large as the area irradiated at 1 foot. At 3 feet, each unit of area, numbered 1 through 9, receives 1/9 of energy as the comparable unit of area at 1 foot. That is, the intensity of radiation is inversely proportional to the square of the distance from the source.

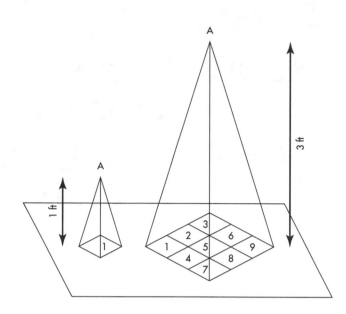

Figure B–1.

$$I \propto \frac{1}{d^2} \quad \text{where: } I = \text{intensity}$$
$$d = \text{distance}$$

It is possible to determine the intensity at a new distance, assuming the angle of incidence is unchanged. Using the example above, if the original intensity (I_1) is known to be 1 unit at 1 foot (d_1), the unknown intensity (I_2) at a new distance of 3 feet (d_2) can be calculated as follows:

It is known that:

$$I_1 \propto \frac{1}{d_1^{\ 2}} \quad \text{and} \quad I_2 \propto \frac{1}{d_2^{\ 2}}$$

Therefore:

$$\frac{I_1}{I_2} = \frac{1/d_1^{\ 2}}{1/d_2^{\ 2}} \quad \text{and} \quad \frac{I_1}{d_2^{\ 2}} = \frac{I_2}{d_1^{\ 2}}$$

Solving for I_2:

$$I_2 = \frac{I_1 d_1^{\ 2}}{d_2^{\ 2}}$$

$$I_2 = \frac{(1)(1)^2}{(3)^2} = \frac{1}{9} \quad \text{unit of light per unit of area at 3 feet}$$

Keeping the energy, E, constant:

$$I_1 t_1 = I_2 t_2$$

Solving for I_2:

$$I_2 = \frac{I_1 t_1}{t_2}$$

It is also known that:

$$I_2 = \frac{I_1 d_1^{\,2}}{d_2^{\,2}}$$

Therefore:

$$\frac{I_1 t_1}{t_2} = \frac{I_1 d_1^{\,2}}{d_2^{\,2}} \quad \text{and} \quad \frac{t_1}{t_2} = \frac{d_1^{\,2}}{d_2^{\,2}}$$

Solving for t_2:

$$t_2 = \frac{t_1 d_2^{\,2}}{d_1^{\,2}}$$

If a patient is receiving 20 minutes of heat from a lamp at 36 in., how long must the treatment be if the lamp is moved to 30 in. and the energy exchange is kept constant?

$t_1 = 20$ min
$d_1 = 36$ in.
$d_2 = 30$ in.
$t_2 = ?$

$$t_2 = \frac{(20)(30)^2}{(36)^2} = 14.6 \text{ min}$$

Cosine Law

The absorption of rays is optimal when they strike the surface on the perpendicular. As the angle between the beam and the perpendicular is increased, efficiency is decreased in proportion to the cosine of that angle.

In a right triangle, the cosine of the angle is defined as the ratio between the side adjacent to the angle and the hypotenuse.

In Figure B–2, Angle A = 0°, and cos A = AB/AB = 1
    Point B receives 100% of the incident radiation.

Figure B-2.

In Figure B–3, Angle A = 30°, and cos A = AB/AC
According to the Pythagorean Theorem,

$$AC = 2, \ CB = 1, \text{ and } AB = \sqrt{3}$$

$$\cos A = \frac{\sqrt{3}}{2} = 0.86$$

The intensity of radiation at Point C is 86% of the incident radiation at Point B.

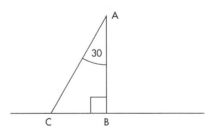

Figure B-3.

In Figure B–4, Angle A = 45°, and cos *A* = *AB/AC*

$$AB = 1, \ CB = 1, \text{ and } AC = \sqrt{2}$$

$$\cos A = \frac{1}{\sqrt{2}} = 0.71$$

The intensity of radiation at Point C is 71% of the incident radiation at Point B.

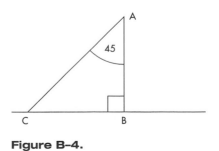

Figure B-4.

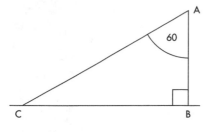

Figure B–5.

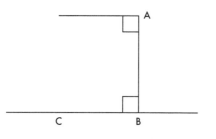

Figure B–6.

In Figure B–5, Angle A = 60°, and cos $A = AB/AC$

$$AB = 1, \ CB = \sqrt{3}, \text{ and } AC = 2$$

$$\cos A = \frac{1}{2} = 0.50$$

The intensity of radiation at Point C is 50% of the incident radiation at Point B.

In Figure B–6, Angle A = 90°, and cos $A = AB/0$ = undefined
Point C receives no energy.

If cosine A represents the percentage of incident radiation that falls on the surface from a beam making an angle, A, with the perpendicular, then

$$I_C = I_B (\cos A)$$

where:

I_B = Intensity at point B
I_C = Intensity at point C

An increase in time would be necessary to compensate for an increase in the angularity of the waves. The increase in time can be calculated. For example, for angle A = 45° (see Figure B–4),

$$I_B t_1 = I_C t_2$$

where:

I_B = 100% or 1.00
I_C = 0.71
t_1 = 1
t_2 = ?

$$t_2 = \frac{I_B t_1}{I_C} = \frac{(1.00)(1)}{0.71} = 1.41$$

Increase the time by 41%.
Table B–1 summarizes the time compensation for the angles discussed.

TABLE B–1. Percentages of Time Compensation for Various Angles of Incidence

ANGLE A° (DEGREES)	% OF INCIDENT RADIATION AT ANGLE A	% TIME INCREASE TO COMPENSATE FOR LOSS OF EFFICIENCY
0	100	0
30	86	16
45	71	41
60	50	100

a At less than 30 degrees, any change in exposure may be overlooked.

Motor Point Charts

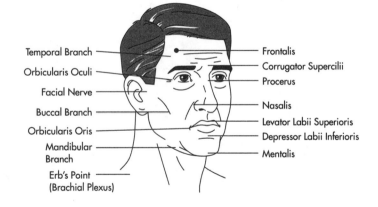

Figure C-1. Motor points of muscles innervated by the facial nerve.

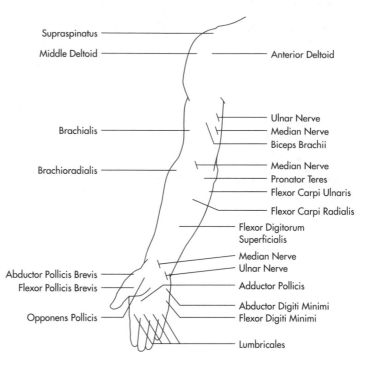

Supraspinatus
Middle Deltoid
Anterior Deltoid
Ulnar Nerve
Brachialis
Median Nerve
Biceps Brachii
Brachioradialis
Median Nerve
Pronator Teres
Flexor Carpi Ulnaris
Flexor Carpi Radialis
Flexor Digitorum Superficialis
Median Nerve
Abductor Pollicis Brevis
Ulnar Nerve
Flexor Pollicis Brevis
Adductor Pollicis
Abductor Digiti Minimi
Opponens Pollicis
Flexor Digiti Minimi
Lumbricales

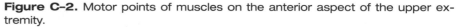

Figure C–2. Motor points of muscles on the anterior aspect of the upper extremity.

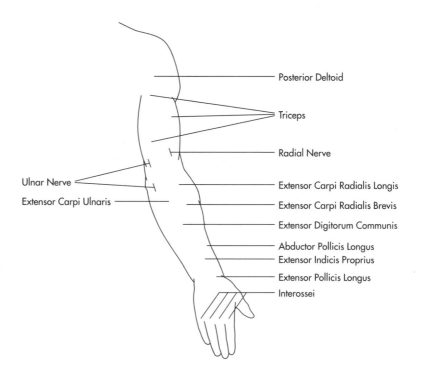

Posterior Deltoid
Triceps
Radial Nerve
Ulnar Nerve
Extensor Carpi Radialis Longis
Extensor Carpi Ulnaris
Extensor Carpi Radialis Brevis
Extensor Digitorum Communis
Abductor Pollicis Longus
Extensor Indicis Proprius
Extensor Pollicis Longus
Interossei

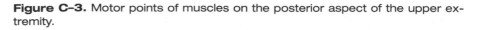

Figure C–3. Motor points of muscles on the posterior aspect of the upper extremity.

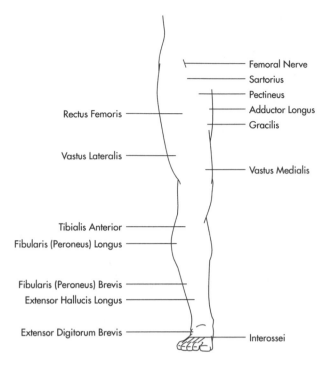

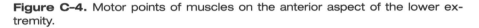

Figure C-4. Motor points of muscles on the anterior aspect of the lower extremity.

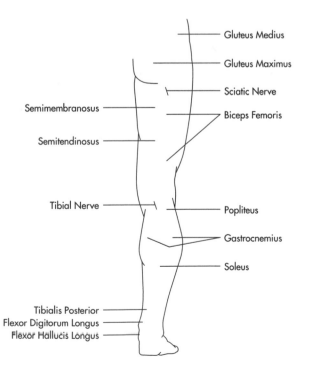

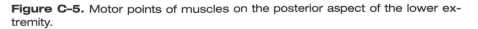

Figure C-5. Motor points of muscles on the posterior aspect of the lower extremity.

Index